**NEW HOLLAND PROFESSIONAL** make-up

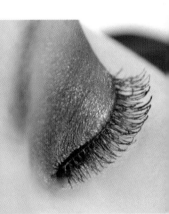

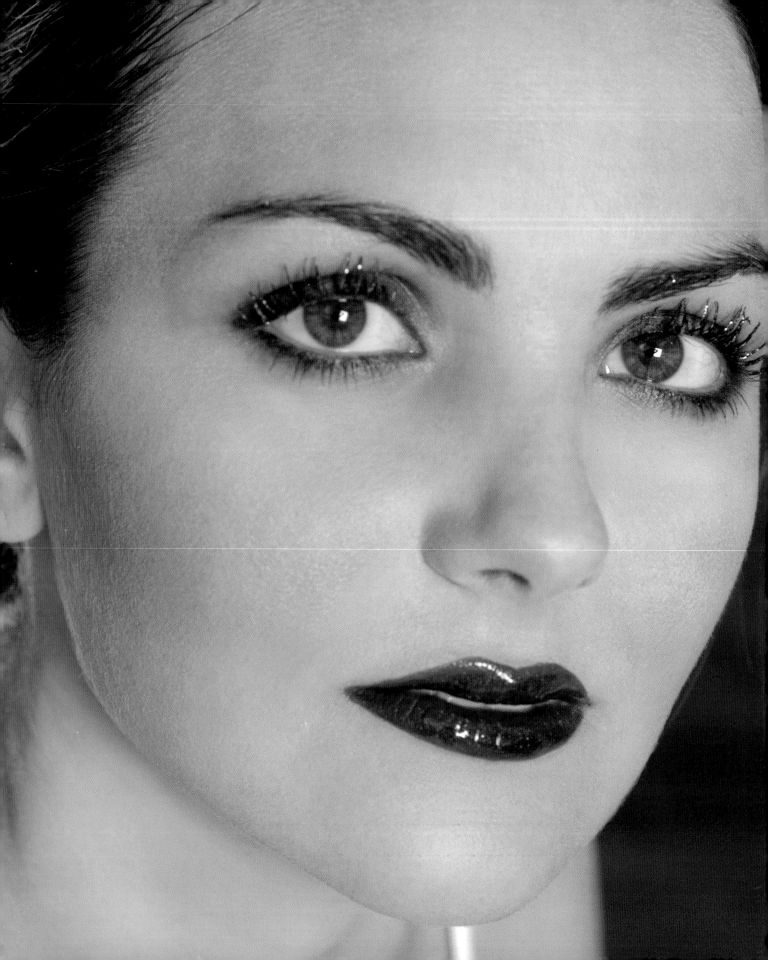

NEW HOLLAND
PROFESSIONAL

# make-up

rosie watson

NEW
HOLLAND

First published in 2007 by New Holland Publishers (UK) Ltd
London • Cape Town • Sydney • Auckland

Garfield House
86-88 Edgware Road
London W2 2EA
United Kingdom
www.newhollandpublishers.com

80 McKenzie Street
Cape Town 8001
South Africa

Unit 1
66 Gibbes Street
Chatswood
NSW 2067
Australia

218 Lake Road
Northcote
Auckland
New Zealand

ISBN  978 1 84537 720 5

Senior Editor **Corinne Masciocchi**
Designer **Lisa Tai**
Photographer **Paul West**
Production **Marion Storz**
Editorial Direction **Rosemary Wilkinson**

10 9 8 7 6 5 4 3 2 1

Reproduction by Pica Digital PTE Ltd, Singapore
Printed and bound by Craft print International Ltd, Singapore

# contents

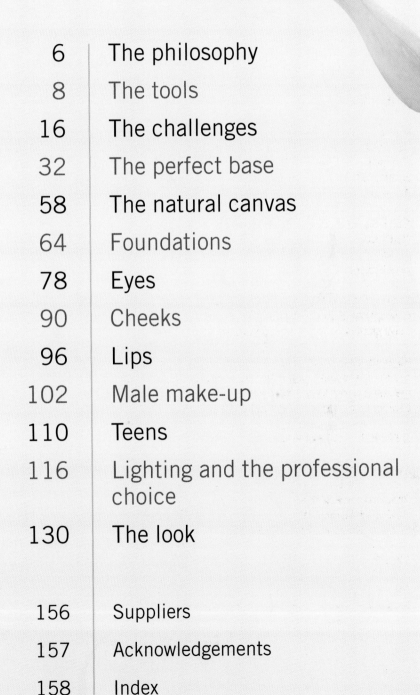

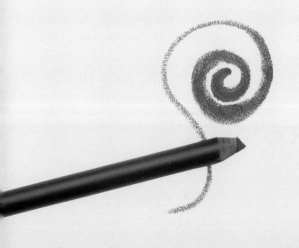

# the philosophy

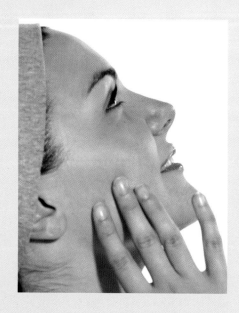

Look in the mirror… there is only one person in the world who looks like you and that is you. Never has a woman looked more beautiful when she is healthy and happy in her own skin. Confidence and self-assurance are wonderful assets, and even if they are not ones you always recognise in yourself or others they can be developed with the aid of make-up. There are no hard and fast rules to make-up application, so experiment with colours and looks until you find a style that suits your or your clients' needs.

A woman should never hide behind a cloak of make-up but rather allow it to enhance her natural beauty and reflect her inner warmth. I have picked up many a golden tip from being surrounded by professional, artistic and creative people throughout my career and this book will hopefully go some way to stimulate you to look at make-up in a more inspiring light.

I always thought make-up was a fashion and that following the pack would make me attractive and trendy. But was I wrong when I tried orange! The art within the art is feeling good about what you wear on your face. So though following the latest trends is not always advisable, make-up should reflect not only someone's personality and mood, but also their lifestyle and wardrobe.

I have chosen to work with 'real' people in this book to illustrate how real beauty can shine through. I have also considered more extravagant ideas but in my eyes they are simple, fantastic ways to manipulate products and tools to give me more make-up options. 'Alright,' I hear you cry, 'there is only one way to apply mascara!' but I will show you there are many ways of wearing it!

In the 1950s people were desperate to get their hands on make-up, as basics such as red lipstick and black eyeliner were pretty much all that was available. In the '60s and '70s experimentation took a back seat, as for the main part single colours were used to exaggerate the eyes with little colour used elsewhere, although make-up trends changed at the end of this era to incorporate nothing but colour. In the '80s and '90s it was just too much of everything, and now in the new millennium you can be as natural or as glamorous as you wish. Never before has there been so much choice and so many varieties of colour, texture, shade and sparkle! As we end this decade, make-up will continue to change and we will see products being invented which will surprise even the most experienced make-up artist. But I look forward to change and hope you do, too.

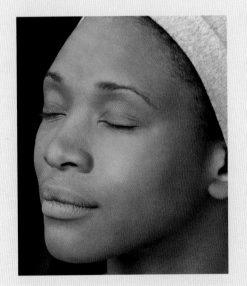

 Never has a woman looked more beautiful when she is healthy and happy in her own skin

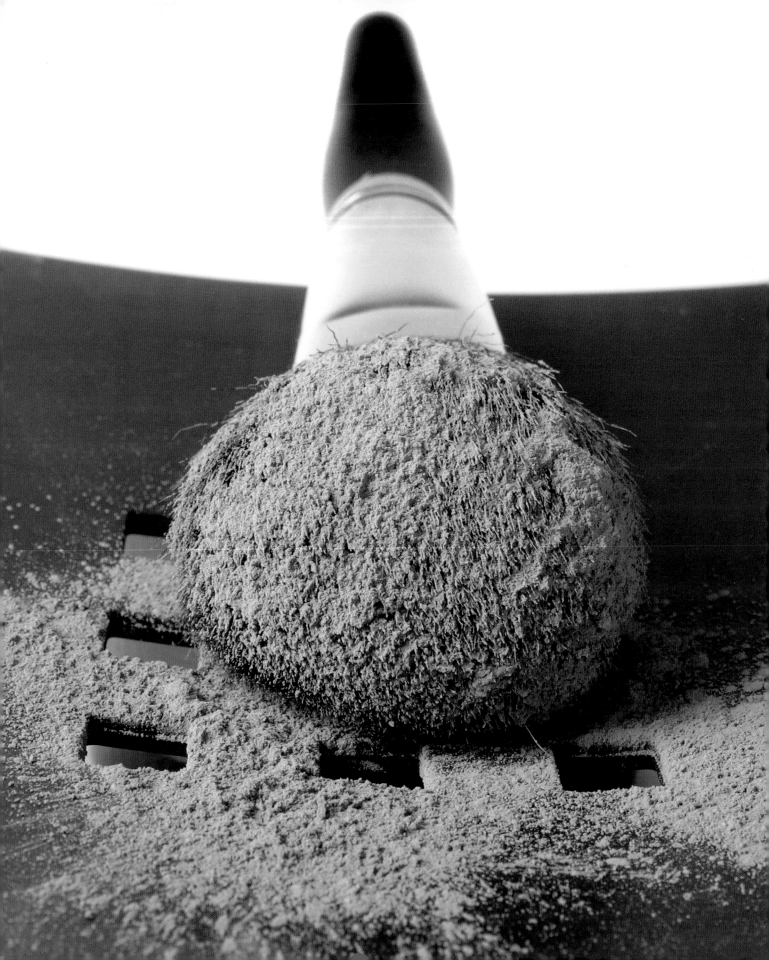

# 01 the tools

# the tools

Precision is what you need for flawless make-up and this can only be achieved with the right tools. Fingertips are a vital part of the tool kit and are your best blenders but getting into small corners with eyeshadow and eyeliner is the job of a suitable brush. The best brushes are soft to the touch and are shaped according to the area of the face being treated. They should be easy to clean and should not release bristles freely.

Both synthetic and natural brushes are readily available and often synthetics are easier to clean, however, the blending power of natural hair in a tightly bound brush is remarkable. The best brushes feel sturdy but are light enough to achieve a feather-like touch to your application. A good set of brushes can easily last years and can prove to be your best investment so choose wisely and always ask to try out the brushes before you buy.

**TYPES OF BRUSHES**
① brow brush
② blending sponge
③ foundation base brush
④ eyeshadow dome
⑤ contour facial brush;
⑥ mini shadow brush
⑦ eyeshadow stubby
⑧ angled eyeliner brush
⑨ angular brow/lash separator
⑩ lip dome
⑪ ⑫ eyeshadow blenders
⑬ blusher brush
⑭ ⑮ powder brush

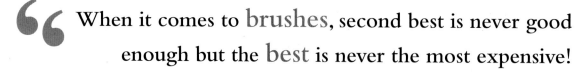

① ② ③ ④ ⑤ ⑥ ⑦ ⑧ ⑨ ⑩ ⑪ ⑫ ⑬ ⑭ ⑮

**When it comes to brushes, second best is never good enough but the best is never the most expensive!**

# Back to basics

Each brush has its own purpose so buy them individually in accordance with the make-up you use on a daily basis. There is no point in wasting money on something you will never use. There are a few essential basics other than brushes, however, which you should include in your kit.

**Lash curlers** The old style is often the best and this is definitely the case with lash curlers! Curled lashes look fantastic with or without make-up as they really open the eyes and give them depth.

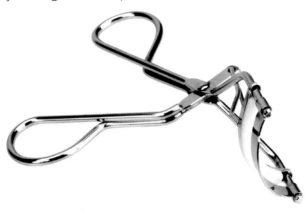

**Sharpener** A good sharpener will have two holes: one for chubby pencils and the other for liners. Finding a good sharpener could save you pounds in shavings! Plastic sharpeners are often better as they are durable and light and are less prone to rust.

**Tweezers** Invest in a good pair of tweezers and carry them with you to pluck out any rogue hairs before venturing out in public! Tweezer tips come in many variations but often slanted or round tips are best as they are easier to handle and great at grabbing hairs.

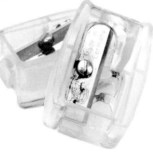

Pointed or flat-tipped versions can prove painful if not used properly as it is often easier to scratch or pinch the skin with these.

**Wedges** You may not use these regularly but when the time comes you'll be glad you invested in them! They are great for blotting, blending and touching up throughout the day. Make sure you change these regularly to avoid spreading any infections and always use your own.

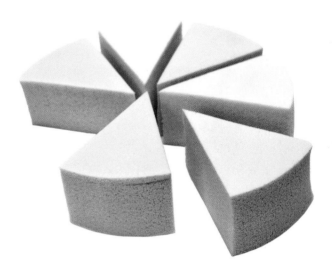

**Cotton buds** Cotton buds are the best tools for removing splodges or mistakes in hard-to-get-to areas and for blending eye pencils if you are missing a brush. Don't be tempted to use the same cotton bud time and again – it should only be used a couple of times before discarding it.

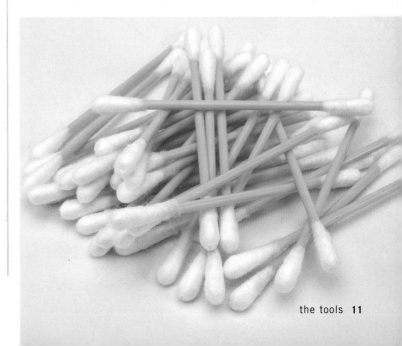

# The tool box

Give an artist one brush and they will paint you a picture but give them a selection and they can create something truly individual with differing textures, strokes and effects. Professional brushes are expected when treating clients but for your home kit you only need invest in a small, but good selection.

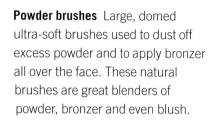

**Powder brushes**  Large, domed ultra-soft brushes used to dust off excess powder and to apply bronzer all over the face. These natural brushes are great blenders of powder, bronzer and even blush.

**Blusher brush**  A smaller domed but still ultra-soft brush which should fit easily on the apple of your cheek without over spreading to prevent too much colour being dropped onto the cheek.

**Powder brushes**

**Foundation base brush**  A medium but flat dome shaped synthetic brush used to apply cream foundation or concealer. This firm brush allows for precision and the ultimate finish.

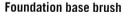
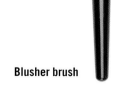

**Blusher brush**

**Foundation base brush**

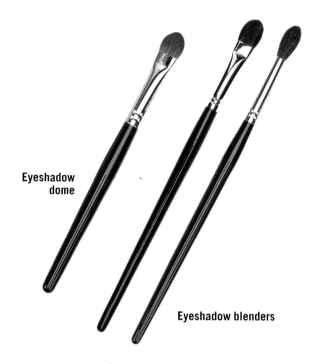

**Eyeshadow dome**

**Eyeshadow blenders**

**Eyeshadow dome**  It is good to have two of these brushes – one for light shadows and one for darker shades. Synthetic brushes are good for precision lines and adding depth to shadows whereas sable brushes, because they are softer, are great for blending and finishing.

**Eyeshadow blenders**  These are very soft, loose-bristle brushes, great for blending blocks or lines of colour as well as smudging light and dark shadows together.

**Eyeshadow stubby**  This square, firm brush is great for dotting on eyeshadow or block liquid liner before blending as it offers high precision.

**Contour facial brush**  This slanted dome brush is great for precision highlighting and shading of the face, especially the cheekbones. A brush like this can be used for practically any purpose so adapt it to fit your every day needs.

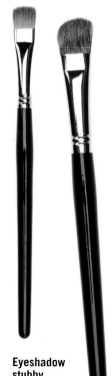

**Eyeshadow stubby**

**Contour facial brush**

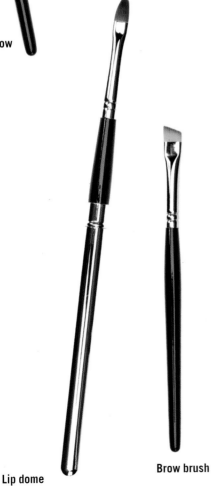

**Mini shadow brush**  This very small dome is great for working along the lashes or close to the eye with shadow as it is firm and enables high precision. It is also a high quality blender, especially effective on lines of dark shadow or liners.

**Lip dome**  This is the main lip brush as it is firm to the touch and lip sized. It is designed to give precision without flooding the lips with colour and enables you to create the perfect lip line.

**Brow brush**  This slanted brush is perfectly designed for contouring eyebrows, as well as applying and blending pencils and eyeshadows. Use the full length of the brush and sweep on the powder. Don't dot or rub the powder on as this will damage the delicate bristles of the brush.

Mini shadow
brush

Lip dome

Brow brush

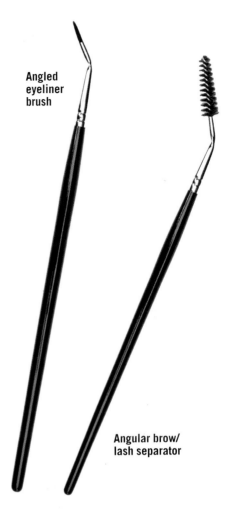

Angled
eyeliner
brush

Angular brow/
lash separator

**Angled eyeliner brush**  This odd looking bent fine line brush is ideally shaped for detailed liquid liner work around the eyes.

**Angular brow/lash separator**  Purposely angled to reach the corners of the lashes and brows to separate and comb the hairs to perfection. Also great for applying clear mascara to these areas. Make sure you clean the brush regularly to prevent the bristles getting clogged up with mascara.

**Blending sponge**  The king of the make-up kit! The blending sponge is superb at blending eyeliner and detailed shadow work around the eyes, as well as just about anything that needs smudging!

Blending sponge

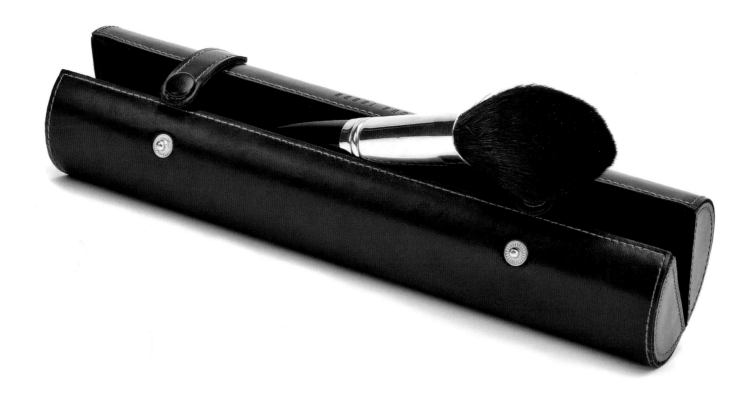

## Storing brushes

Professional make-up artists insist on using the correct brush for specific areas of the face as it makes their job easier. The packs of sponge applicators from the chemist are fine but to really gain precision and increase your artistry buy professional brushes and see the difference. We quite often spend an incredible amount of money on make-up products but aren't bothered about applying them properly!

Take care of your brushes and store them in a pouch, roll or box designed to keep them safe and away from dust and possible damage.

To prevent brush damage and cross contamination ensure you clean your brushes well after every use. Brushes house microbes and bacteria which can cause infections and skin rashes if not kept meticulously clean.

## trade tips

### FOR BRUSHES

- Always try out the brushes you want to buy first by brushing them against the back of your hand and making sure the bristles do not fall out.

- Make sure you buy a proprietary brush cleaner as although soap and warm water are an option they can leave a scum residue on the brush fibres, which can cause clogging and concentration of colour. Brush cleaner contains mild alcohols that dissolve grease and any build up of cosmetics on the brush fibres.

- Brushes should be firm but flexible and have an even spread of bristles when pressure is applied.

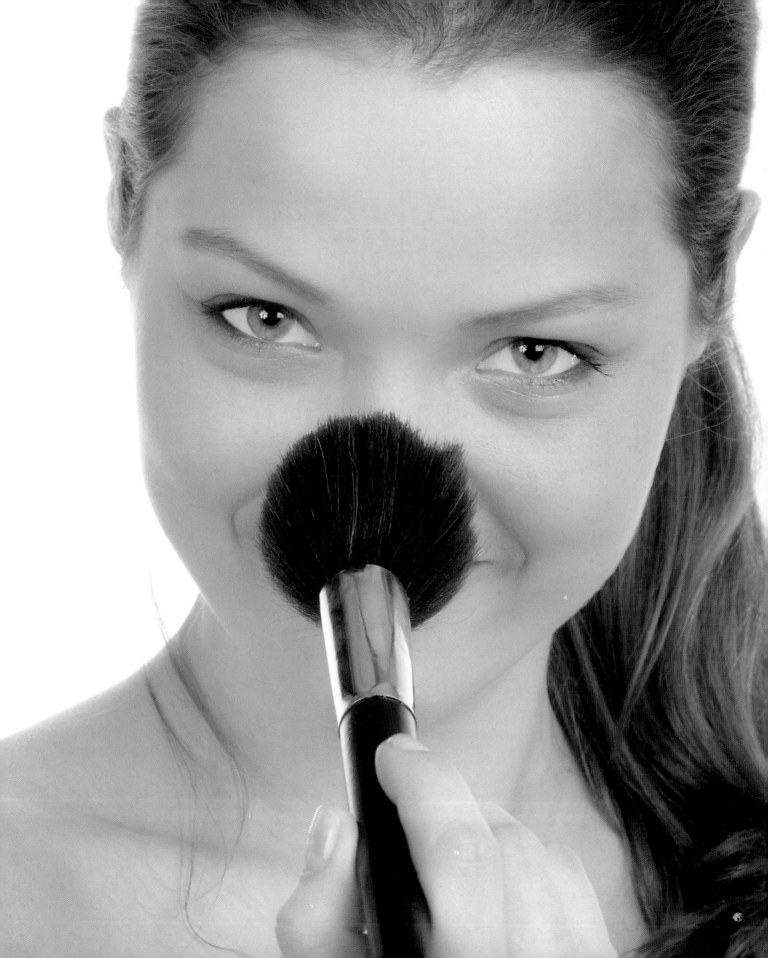

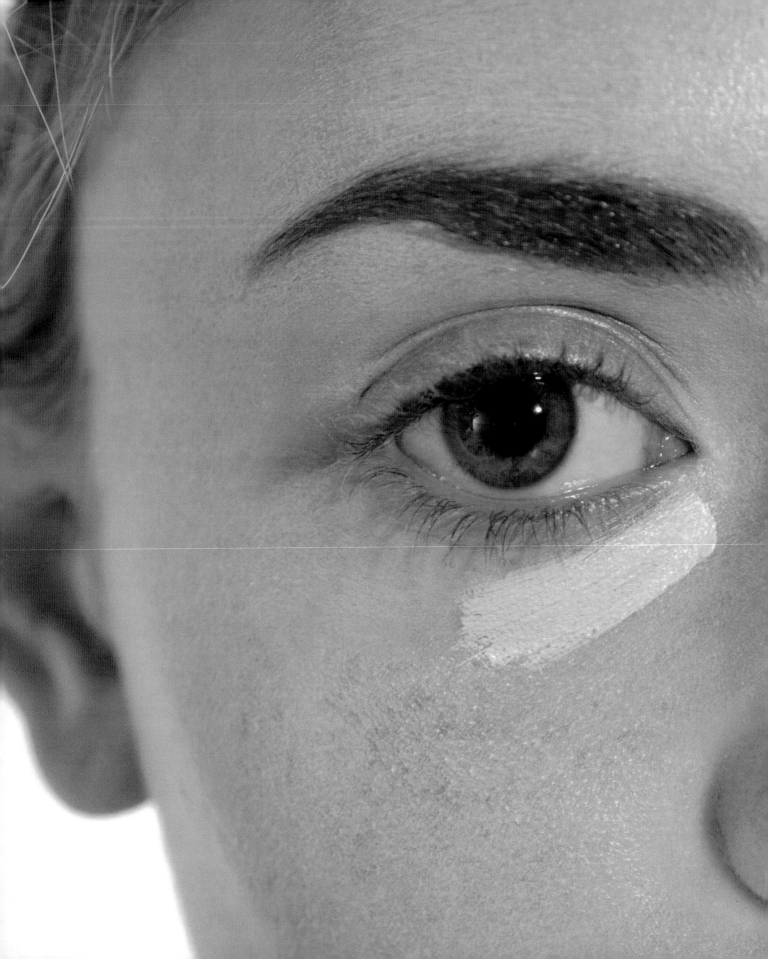

# 02 the challenges

# the challenges

Every make-up assignment has its own challenges and the process of overcoming them is extremely rewarding. Not every skin has a smooth, creamy appearance and not everyone has model features but with proper application, make-up can transform features, softening the ones you don't like so much and emphasising the ones you do. There is nothing more satisfying than making the best of someone's natural features and often people can become incredibly emotional when they see their transformation after make-up.

 Make up can be a reflection of inner expression or an emotional fortification

## Skin reading

Not all skins tolerate make-up because they are 'contra-indicated' to treatment. This means that applying make-up could be harmful, either because the skin is damaged or because it is susceptible to an allergic reaction. Read your skin's external messages and decide if you need to make changes to your make-up to make its application safe and comfortable.

## Sensitive skins

Sensitivity can frequently occur when using skin preparations and make-up. Itching, swelling, excess heat, stinging and irritation are common reactions to products that contain perfume, alcohol and preservatives. Protect sensitive skin with an underbase (primer) product which is applied over moisturiser and acts as a barrier to protect your skin from harsh ingredients.

## Watch out for changes

Your skin changes regularly to help protect against the environment, pollutants and extremes in temperature, as well as mirroring your internal health and wellbeing. Change your routine when necessary to treat the skin you have. Often the moisturiser or foundation you use in the summer is of too light a consistency and too dark a colour for winter usage. Coverage and colours change during the year as your skin changes colour so be flexible and adapt your skincare and make-up routine. If any unusual skin changes occur during the year you should consult your doctor or a dermatologist. The sun can encourage lesions, along with growth and pigmentation irregularities so for peace of mind have a regular skin check-up.

## Hyper pigmentation

Skin pigmentation disorders occur because the body produces either too much or too little melanin, a pigment that creates hair and skin colour. On light skins, hyper pigmentation manifests itself as small patches of darker skin and on darker skins lighter patches can occur. Make-up can be applied over these areas and a heavier concealer in your natural skin shade can balance colour changes on your face.

Many skin conditions can also be treated with make-up but as a make-up artist you will need to know how to identify them so you can make an educated decision on whether it is safe and comfortable for the client to continue. You may think it is alright to cover a cold sore but when you get three in its place you might be unpleasantly surprised! If in doubt, don't risk it. Get any skin changes checked by a doctor or dermatologist.

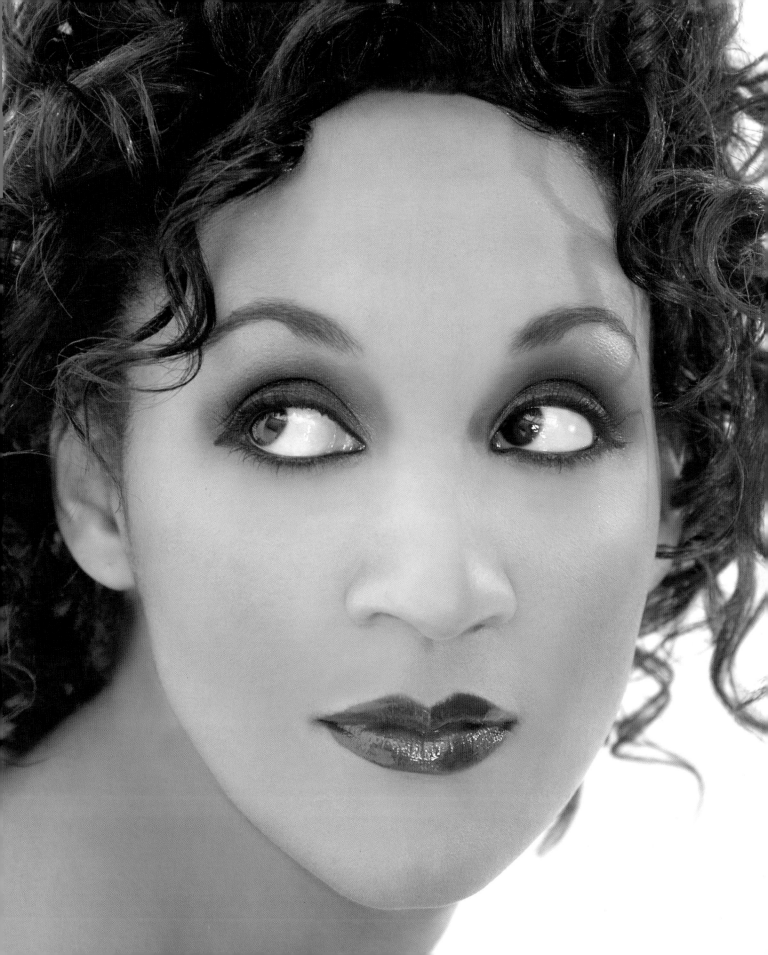

# Problematic pigmentation

Cloasma, vitiligo, lentigo and port wine stains are all common pigmentation irregularities. They appear as discolouration to the face, usually brown or pink in appearance, and can be covered with make-up using camouflage techniques to even the skin's texture and colour.

# Battling bacteria

Boils, sties, conjunctivitis and impetigo are all forms of bacterial infection which can affect make-up application. Most are contagious and infectious so a doctor's advice is needed before applying make-up to prevent cross-infection to yourself and others.

# Viral infections

Cold sores, shingles, warts and verrucas are all viral infections which are extremely difficult to get rid of as the virus stays in the body for years, often a lifetime, resurfacing during times of stress or low immunity. Make-up should be avoided where possible to prevent cross infection of the surrounding skin.

# Fungal infections

Tinea (ringworm) appears as red scaly patches of dry skin and can affect the face, head, feet, hands and nails. Always consult a doctor before applying make-up over these areas as tinea is highly contagious and can cross-infect other areas of the body very easily.

# Skin disorders

Long-term skin complaints such as eczema, which originates from the blood stream, dermatitis, from external sources such as jewellery, and psoriasis can be traumatic to live with and the symptoms vary from dry flaky skin to open wounds, bleeding and itching. In some cases the cause of these conditions is unknown, however, most sufferers say that stress, anxiety and a lack of well-being contributes to a bout. Make-up can be applied but if the skin is sore it is better to let it heal naturally.

Camouflage make-up, such as thick foundations and concealers which block out colour and irregularities on the skin, give the appearance of an even tone. Pick products that are exactly the same as your skin tone and base and use both to eradicate uneven pigmentation. This make-up works wonders on darker birthmarks like port wine stains or strawberry marks. If you want to diminish redness follow the usual concealing rules but use this unique thick consistency make-up instead.

# Cross infection

Every day we lose millions of skin cells and hair strands, and we perspire many hundreds of millilitres of sweat – we just can't see it up close. I never consider using other make-up artists' brushes and they would not ask to borrow mine. It is responsible and professional to never leave yourself liable for cross infection of bacteria or viruses.

Brush cleaning products go some way to cleansing the used make-up and bacteria from your brushes but be aware

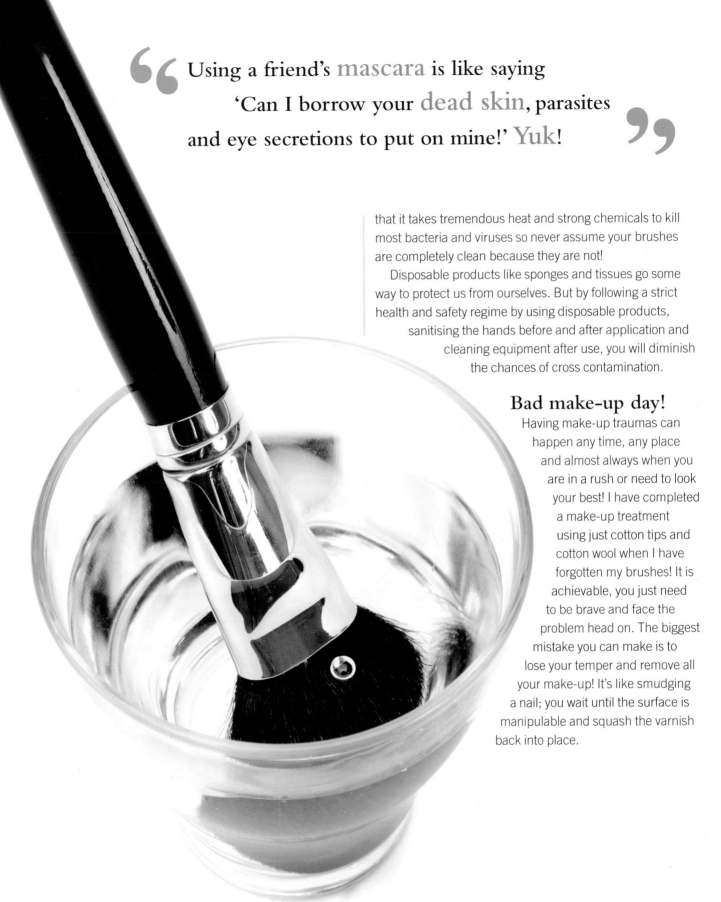

> "Using a friend's mascara is like saying 'Can I borrow your dead skin, parasites and eye secretions to put on mine!' Yuk!"

that it takes tremendous heat and strong chemicals to kill most bacteria and viruses so never assume your brushes are completely clean because they are not!

Disposable products like sponges and tissues go some way to protect us from ourselves. But by following a strict health and safety regime by using disposable products, sanitising the hands before and after application and cleaning equipment after use, you will diminish the chances of cross contamination.

### Bad make-up day!

Having make-up traumas can happen any time, any place and almost always when you are in a rush or need to look your best! I have completed a make-up treatment using just cotton tips and cotton wool when I have forgotten my brushes! It is achievable, you just need to be brave and face the problem head on. The biggest mistake you can make is to lose your temper and remove all your make-up! It's like smudging a nail; you wait until the surface is manipulable and squash the varnish back into place.

# Everyday problems

There are measures to combat any problem and hopefully these tips will help:

**Perspiration** When you are in a rush or a panic the last thing you need is for make-up to be difficult to apply because you are too hot and flustered, so find a window or a fan and try to externally cool yourself. Water evaporates quickly so any extra air flow will help remove excess water from your face.

Blot away excess perspiration – never wipe it off or you will remove the make-up. Spritzing your face provides a much needed cooling effect and removes the salt which is found in sweat to give your skin a fresh look and feel.

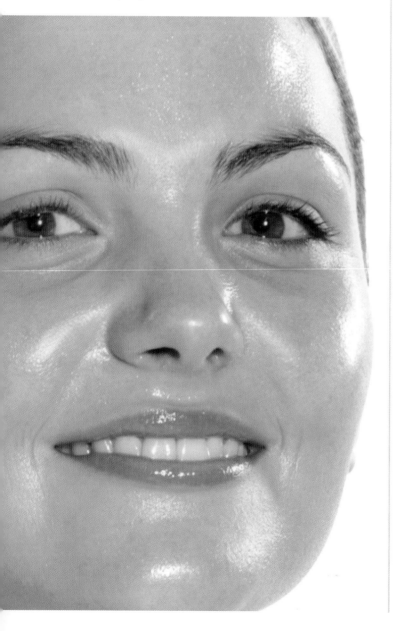

**Blemishes** can be the bane of your life and make-up rarely sticks to a shiny blemish. Use a wax-based skin-coloured concealer to cover the redness but apply it with a cotton tip as the warmth from your fingers will spread the product too much. Apply powder to seal the concealer and this should give you a paler, less noticeable surface. If all else fails cover with normal foundation and tell everyone you are still young enough to get spots!

Never pick a spot before applying make-up as it will weep and the bacteria within could spread. Filling the hole from a picked spot is not the best option as it will inevitably give you another blemish!

**Uneven make-up** can look awful because your skin is not evenly textured or has a diverse moisture content. Following a good skincare routine and moisturising just prior to make-up will do the trick. A flawless surface can be achieved if you use an underbase primer product to mattify the skin prior to make-up application.

# Anti mature

Because of pressures to look younger for longer many of us are turning to anti-ageing treatments in an attempt to prolong a youthful appearance. The market for these types of product is huge – and confusing at times – what with medical cosmetic treatments available as well as those from beauty salons and the shop shelf. So, what should you choose?

There are a number of natural products that can be used both externally and internally to boost the skin's regeneration capabilities, but first let's look at how skin is affected by the daily pressures of modern life.

### FREE RADICALS

Free radicals are disturbed oxygen molecules that are damaging to the skin and to the inner workings of the body. They are caused mainly by UV radiation from the sun, stress, obesity, smoking, pollution and chemical additives.

A healthy body is able to cope with regular attacks from free radicals but if there is over-exposure to one or more of the factors listed above, the body starts to degenerate. One of the early visible symptoms is a change in the skin's appearance. The skin will start to sag and wrinkle at a much earlier stage. So how much are we actively accelerating the process with the way we live our lives?

We can defend ourselves from these free radical scavengers by increasing our exposure to antioxidants. These are chemical compounds that have a reparative effect and destroy the damage caused by the free radicals. Antioxidants can be found naturally in vitamins A, C and E and often make-up artists will use these topically on the skin to encourage an even texture.

We know that unprotected over-exposure to the sun causes skin ailments and using an SPF of at least 15 every day is essential in battling free radicals and maintaining youthful skin. The skin absorbs the sun's strong UV rays and in the process warps and damages cells which can, over time, be the cause of skin cancers.

Eating pre-packaged foods and foods containing artificial colours and preservatives again increases your intake of radicals and will reflect badly on your skin, increasing dryness and encouraging cellular breakdown, leading to obvious lines and wrinkles.

Green tea, herbal or fruit extracts, are natural extracts added to cosmetics. They are natural antioxidants that work to protect the skin from UVB sun rays – the rays that cause the skin to burn when exposed to them. In turn this damaged skin will reduce its production of collagen and consequently increase wrinkle production, so taking preventative steps will reduce the effects of these harmful rays.

▶ *Nature's fusion of fruit, herb or plant extracts enhance the anti-oxidant power of cosmetics.*

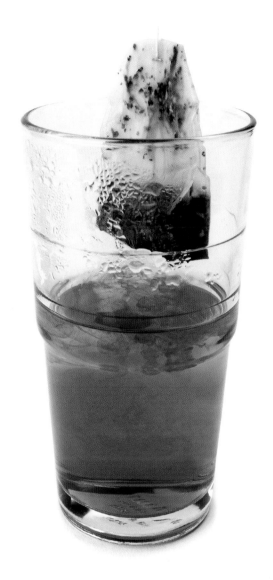

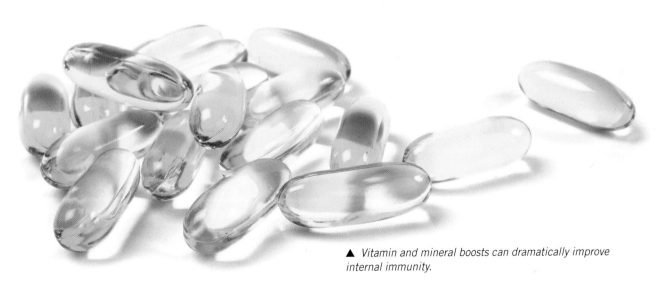

▲ *Vitamin and mineral boosts can dramatically improve internal immunity.*

# "Live life through your skin – don't hide behind it! "

## Juicy genetics

You are quite simply half your mother and half your father so the easiest place to look for clarification on how you will look when you are older is directly at them! Some improvement can be made by reducing radical damage throughout your life, so fear not!

People with good skin genetics are few and far between. Most of us have to work a little to get the results we want from our skin and often we are still not satisfied. Therefore, resorting to chemical and surgical intervention, which provides immediate results, suits many people.

Nowadays, more and more of us are going under the needle or knife to change our appearance. Genetically you are what you are and living with that should place realistic boundaries on what you can and cannot achieve with your looks. Some people continue to change themselves with surgery either to create a totally new look or to try to balance some internal hardship.

Genetics can be cruel or wonderful but the skin you are in is what you have to work with so being realistic will save you getting anxious about your skin and stimulating the need for change.

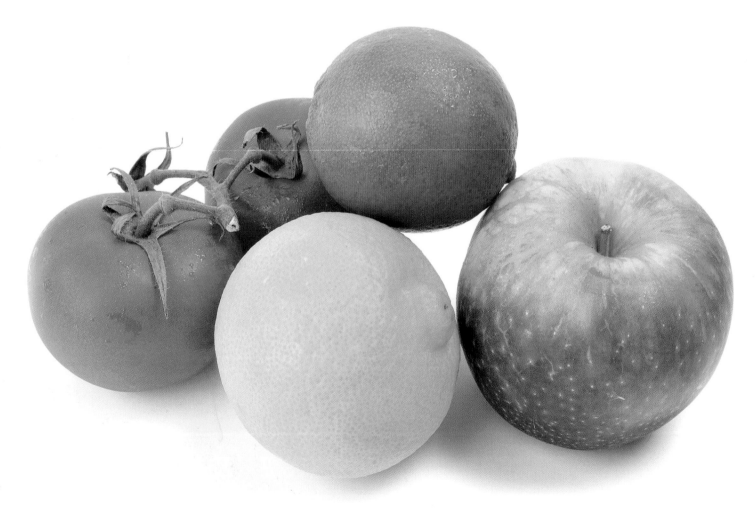

# Fabulous future

Some swear by them while others wouldn't touch them with a barge pole. Anti-ageing products are continually being developed to help overcome our ageing concerns. Give them a try and see if you notice a difference but I wouldn't recommend attempting a skin peel or dermabrasion yourself at home – even though there are many products available, they are manufactured to be substantially weaker than professional products and the results can therefore be mediocre! This should be left to the professionals.

## SOME OF THE CURRENT KEY INGREDIENTS IN THE MATURE MARKET ARE:

★ **Co Enzyme Q10** Used to boost energy within a skin cell and to promote rejuvenation of healthy cells. It is also a powerful antioxidant that prevents free radical damage to the skin cells' energy centres. This is a chemical compound and there is no evidence that currently suggests how deep the ingredients penetrate into the skin, however, Q10 is also found in our bodies naturally and dietary supplements such as liver, kidney, beef, soy oil, sardines, mackerel, and peanuts all help to maintain diminishing amounts as we get older. By utilising a product both internally and externally the effects could be doubled!

★ **Hyaluronic acid** An acid that holds 1000 times its weight in water and when used on the skin provides super hydration qualities. It is found in the dermis and helps maintain collagen and elastin in the skin. We have a great deal of naturally occurring HA in our body when we are born but with age this diminishes and soft, smooth skin is harder to achieve. HA can be used topically and is often added to cosmetic creams or ingested in tablet form.

★ **Vitamin A** Is a skin softening and resurfacing product used topically on the skin in cream, lotion or liquid forms. Retinoids, derived from vitamin A, all have common results. Retinyl palmitate makes up the highest portion of vitamin A found in the skin and is the least known skin irritant of the vitamin A family. It gives the skin a smoother and softer appearance, reducing the signs of ageing by relaxing wrinkles and plumping the skin. Anti-ageing vitamin A treatments are available over the counter and offer a much needed boost to the naturally diminishing amounts in the body as we age.

★ **Ascorbic acid** Also known as vitamin C. Unfortunately for our skin, vitamin C quickly degenerates on contact with oxygen so vitamin C cosmetics tend to be very expensive due to the stabilising products needed to stop the vitamin going off. Ascorbic acid and other Vitamin C derivatives are good for anti-ageing because they have an exfoliation action as well as one which synthesises collagen production and maintains good amounts of flexibility in the skin.

Prevention is better than cure and many treatments are now available, from facial exercising to multi-step facial programmes. Equally you can home prepare facial treatments to help combat anti-ageing and using simple mixtures of vitamins A, C and E in a face mask will really help freshen your face. Experiment with different combinations and textures before buying expensive alternatives and if you can, ask a dermatologist what will work best for you.

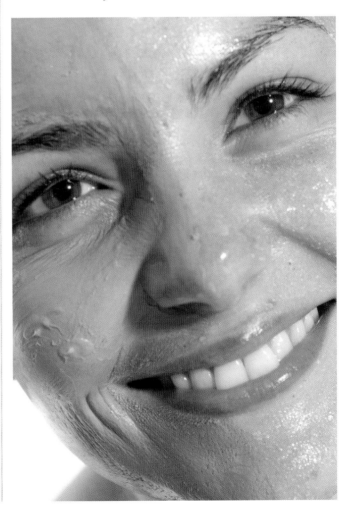

# Skin expectations

Ageing of the skin starts at around the age of 21 because the skin cell reproduction process slows. So what should we expect? What is natural and happens to us all? Although genetically you will have the same skin as your parents, it is possible to appear younger over time, especially by making sure you use adequate sun protection, and cleanse and moisturise your skin regularly.

# 15s

## TEENS

Below the age of 20 but during puberty the skin is constantly adjusting to the surge of hormones that help us develop into young adults. Skin changes can vary but often an increased oil production makes the skin spotty and shiny. The skin is at its peak here and everything inside it is functioning well and to its limit. Although this can be a difficult time, especially if you suffer from acne, treat it well. It is important to protect the skin from over-exposure to the sun and to try not to pick spots as this will encourage bacteria to spread on the skin causing more spots and sometimes permanent scarring.

Tea tree products offer a good solution as they are blemish treatments but also make you feel fresh and smell nice! All skins should first be cleansed and then moisturised with a minimum SPF of 15. If out in the sun, don't plaster your skin with baby oil for a fast tan – the damage you do now to the dermis will remain with you forever and you will age much faster!

# 20s

## TWENTIES

Your skin is still 'young' at this stage but has already begun to age and some fine expression lines may begin to appear in the mid- to late-twenties due to small amounts of collagen diminishing in the skin. Mild pigmentation can also occur due to sun damage, and the use of harsh products like alcohols, perfumes, preservatives and colours can lead to sensitivity in this stage of our lives.

A regular facial will work wonders as it will support the skin's mechanisms whilst boosting cell reproduction. The eye area will need extra attention in the form of a light gel or cream to help nourish and prevent deepening of lines. Always cleanse, tone and moisturise with an SPF of 15 mornings and evenings, especially when wearing make-up, and be sure to incorporate the neck with your daily nourish. Hands should also be treated daily with a rich hand cream and avoid harsh chemical products on the skin as once sensitised, the skin can stay that way.

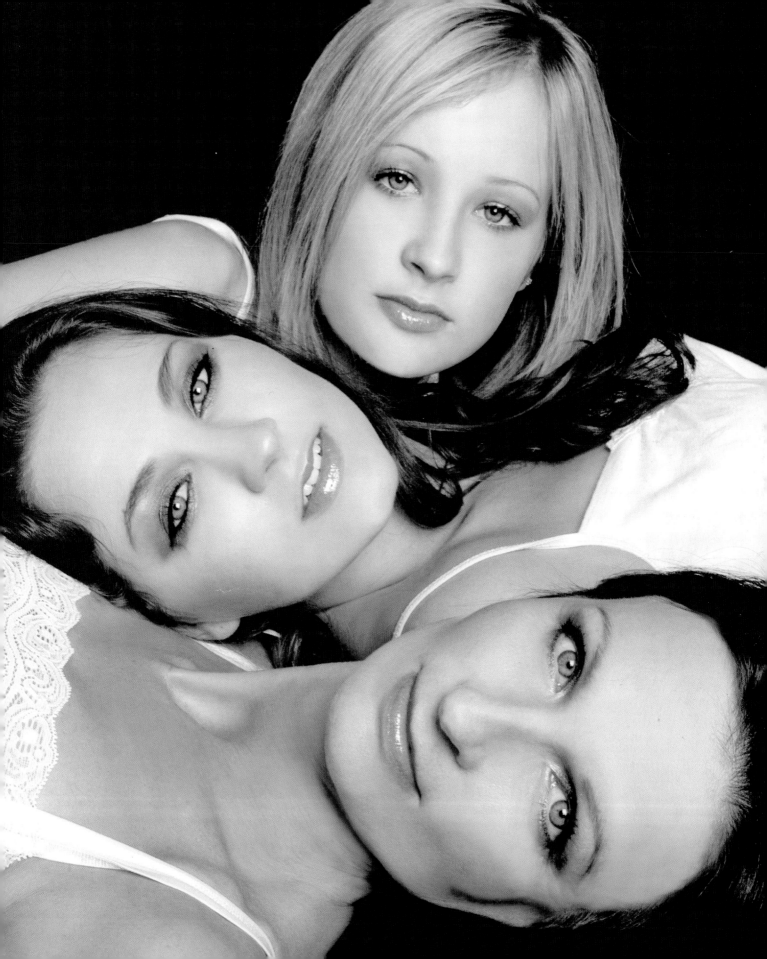

# 30s

## THIRTIES

Most of the possible damage to the skin by the sun has already occurred at this stage but it will not show until later in life so treat your skin well now to reduce the appearance of damage later. Age spots may start to show along with some pigmentation changes from the sun. Mainly though, the skin will continue to lose collagen and elastin, giving the skin a lack of plumpness and increasing the risk of sagging muscle tone and dryness.

Adults in their 30s can still suffer from oily skin but this is rare as the hormones responsible have balanced themselves. However, it has been proven that stress and pregnancy can trigger an outburst. Lines and wrinkles will appear much deeper now and dehydration is a regular occurrence.

Regular facial treatments with your therapist or at home will help stimulate the skin cells, and topical skin ingredients such as natural extracts found in moisturisers can go some way to preventing further damage from the sun and free radicals.

# 40s

## FORTIES

During this time the skin will rapidly continue to show signs of ageing if not properly taken care of. Sun protection is now vital to prevent moles and blemishes changing into cancerous lesions. Sebum production is dramatically reduced, leading to the deepening of lines and wrinkles. Dryness, enlarged pores, deepening discolouration under the eyes and an increase in thread veins (broken capillaries) on the cheeks all start to rear their ugly head.

The full spectrum of cosmetics can be used, such as eye creams and masks as well as a good exfoliation on a weekly basis to remove dead cells that give skin a flaky or dull appearance. This is the age when chemical peels and surgical treatments are mostly carried out as the skin really shows clear signs of ageing. But looking after your skin as best you can and learning to accept the inevitable ageing process will help you feel happier and more comfortable with it.

# 50s

## FIFTIES

The skin is now very different to that of younger years, having more lines and wrinkles as well as deeper furrows around the mouth. The skin sags in places and lack of muscle tone makes the skin appear drawn. The skin is usually dryer at this age but with the onset of the menopause and the subsequent hormonal changes, adult acne can sometimes occur due to the increase in fluctuating hormones, and appears just as in teenage acne with the skin becoming excessively oily and spotty. Skin can become uneven so along with a good regular facial routine and treatments from the therapist, exfoliate regularly to help regulate the surface texture. Broken capillaries and age spots should be expected but be sure to sun protect as ever to help prevent further dermis damage.

Anti-ageing creams and lotions are mostly used in this stage of life but a healthy diet and regular exercise are essential to keep the skin healthy and young looking.

Above all skincare should be fun and not an obsession. Remember that stress is a major ager so staying healthy on the inside and out and stress-free in the shade is the best way forward!

## Anti-mature make-up!

Disguising skin changes can be really effective and easy. With every skin change ageing inflicts there is a solution to combat it with make-up!

**Dry skin**  Use a good moisturiser and primer under your make-up to mattify the skin and remove all traces of uneven patches of dryness whilst preventing make-up sinking into flaky, uneven skin. Follow with a light tinted foundation to give a sheer coverage and a light-reflective appearance.

**Lines and wrinkles**  Use products that don't sink into creases around the eyes. Light and powder-based eyeshadows work best. Avoid shine and shimmer as these exaggerate ageing effects. Cream shadows look great for the cheeks. Using facial, lip and eye primers will go some way to preventing make-up seeping in so apply those before the foundation.

**Thin skin**  This type of skin can look radiant but if you don't like the effect increase your foundation coverage slightly and apply natural shades of blush and bronzer to add a healthy glow to possible sallow skin.

**Saggy skin**  Facial contouring to shade and highlight areas of the face are a nice idea and using light-reflective foundations draws attention away from saggy skin. Light, bright colours are great on eyes and lips but always go natural with blush.

**Hot flush!**  At times of extreme heat remember to blot and not wipe away excess perspiration and try to use a foundation which is fairly low coverage so pores do not show during the day. Try a peachy blush or bronzer rather than red tones as the skin will flush these anyway.

**Droopy eyes**  Use a light colour eyeshadow all over the lid to open the eye area and stick to natural colours. Avoid shimmer and shine at all costs! Never use liquid liner as it tends to splodge onto the lid; opt for a smoky eye pencil instead. Curl the eyelashes and follow with a lighter shade of mascara as it is not so harsh.

**Deteriorating lips**  Use a primer base to prevent lipstick bleeding and choose a matt lipstick in your preferred shade. Add gloss if you like but wet lips can look odd on lips of age so a shimmer will be more flattering.

# how to...

## REVERSE TIME WITH MAKE-UP

Although skin faces many challenges with age we can certainly appear to reverse time with make-up. Light and subtle shades and shimmers create a natural but glowing youth which complements any age and any skin identity.

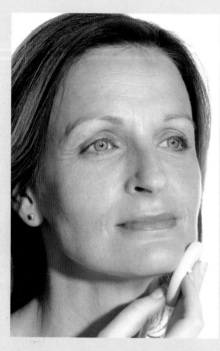

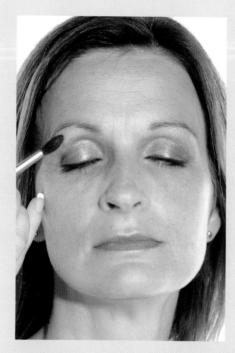

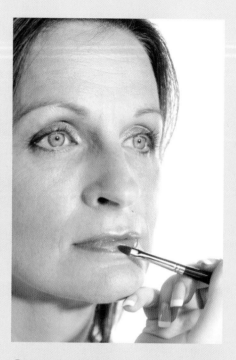

① Apply a light foundation with light-reflective properties so it never looks powdery. Conceal the areas of concern but avoid concealing under the eyes with a heavy wax-based concealer as this may run into the fine lines around the eyes and draw unwanted attention. Choose a liquid concealer instead.

② Using a cream champagne coloured eyeshadow will open the eyes and highlight under the brow for more definition. Plucking rogue hairs from the brows will lift the arch and open the eyes.

③ Curl the lashes and apply a grey or brown mascara to complete the natural look. Eyeliner pencil looks great to define the corners of the eyes and to widen them. Apply a pink or peach blush to the apples of the cheeks and blend to look natural. Lip primer and liner will provide the best base for lipstick. Apply a matt colour to the lips adding sheer shimmer to the centre of the lips for an evening look.

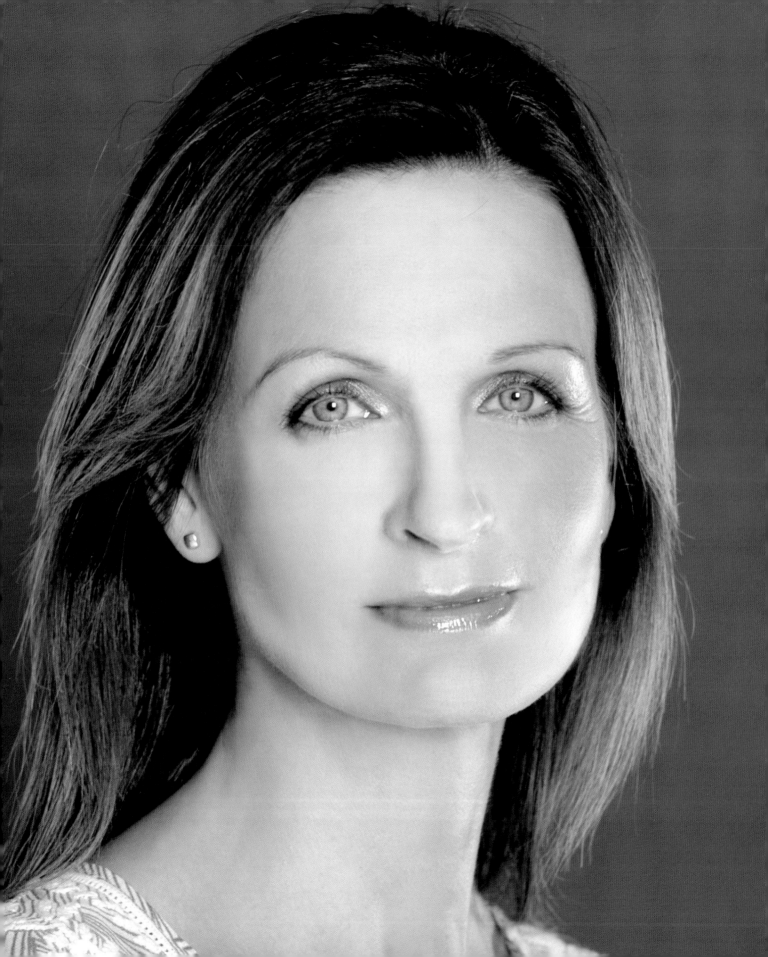

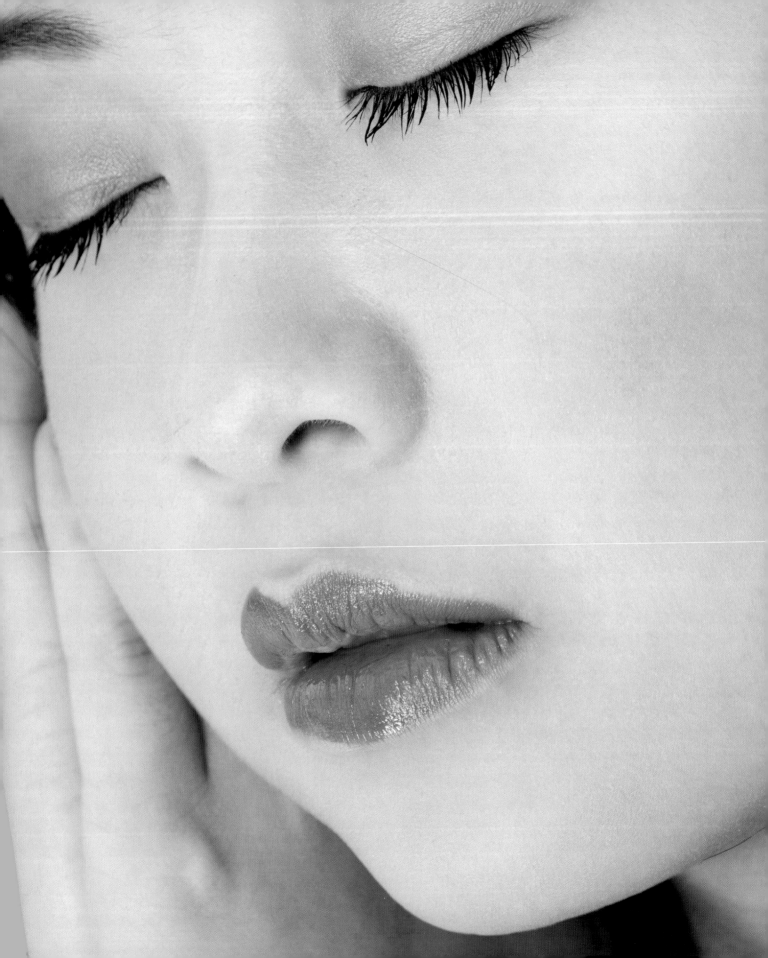

# 03 the perfect base

# the perfect base

As the largest organ in the body, the skin weighs around 3 kg (7 lb) and has a huge role to play in maintaining our health, protecting delicate areas of the body and helping us rid our body of toxins and bacteria. Regardless of what your skin looks like you can always improve its appearance.

Unlike any other organ in the body the skin literally ages before our eyes and the modern day woman is pressured into looking youthful, plucked, pouting and perfect day and night. But unless you are born with beautiful skin genetics passed on from your parents this can be a hard task, especially as everything we look at in the mirror is already made of purely dead cells! My advice therefore is do the best you can with the skin that covers you and be realistic!

The beauty industry is worth billions each year and we are all desperate to conform to the ideal. But let's first feel comfortable in our own skin. Small steps promote a healthy glow and allow skin to appear fresher and radiant, naturally.

Make-up was invented to cover up features we do not like and to accentuate those we do. By improving the skin as a base you will inevitably improve the finished result of your make-up artistry.

Nowhere gets more attention with cosmetics than your face. This is the part of the body people will immediately see and speak to; it shows emotion and can be very easy to read. It is usually the only area we regularly apply make-up to and is the most expressive part of the body. It allows us to show passion, anger, hatred and joy. Make-up should therefore complement our expressions not hide them.

## Skin close up and personal

The skin comprises three layers, the first of which is the surface epidermis, which is paper thin and contains mainly dead or dying skin cells. The next layer is called the dermis and is about 15 times thicker and contains collagen, elastin and a blood supply to feed and nourish the skin. Finally the subcutaneous layer is a layer of insulating fat to keep us warm and protected.

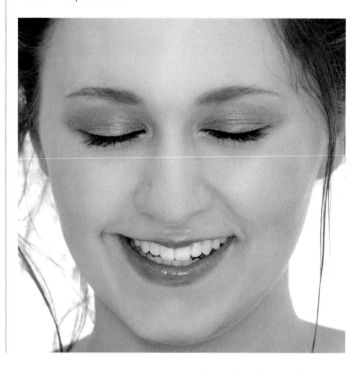

" The skin depicts every emotion you have ever had in its lines, wrinkles and texture; beauty may be skin deep but the skin tells tales, showing all who gaze onto it the story of our lives "

## THE SKIN AND ITS SECTION

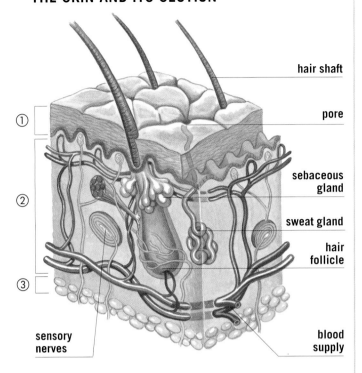

hair shaft

pore

sebaceous gland

sweat gland

hair follicle

sensory nerves

blood supply

▲ ① epidermis (true skin covering)
② dermis (true skin)
③ subcutaneous layer (fat layer)

## SKIN FACTS

- The skin is fed with oxygen, water and nutrients by the blood circulating in the dermis. The epidermis consists of five layers, with the top three made of dead or dying cells.

- Sebum, the skin's natural oil, gives the skin its suppleness. It also provides a sticky surface for bacteria to get caught in. If we do not clean the skin properly this bacteria can build up and infect pores or hair follicles, causing blemishes.

- Blushing is caused by the nervous system triggering a response to emotion which stimulates the blood to rush to the surface of the skin and appears as red or even purple skin tones.

- Free radicals such as the sun's UV rays and oxygen cause dramatic skin ageing.

- Skin is make of the same substances as nails and hair, which is why it is so strong.

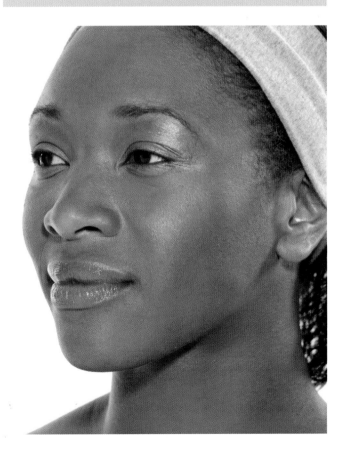

# Skin ID

Identifying your skin's needs helps you decide what products to use and in what quantities to help it reach its full glowing potential. Many make the mistake of misidentifying our skin type and subsequently our treatment of it. The best time of day to decide your skin identity is in the morning when you have allowed the sebum zones to fill with this natural oil from the sebaceous glands in the skin. Sebum is great for protecting the skin against bacteria and pollutants as well as making it soft and supple. However, too much sebum can cause skin blockages and that shiny look we are so desperate to get rid of.

Most of us have combination skin as very few people will have the same exact skin texture, look and feel in all areas of the face. If you are one of the fortunate few, this is described as 'normal skin' – I prefer to call it miracle skin! Treat the problem areas of your skin first as this will balance and blend the problematic patches and give an even look to your complexion.

# Dry skin identification

Dry skin is often found in older or mature skin as over the years sebum production is greatly reduced, opening the skin to the ravages of pollution and ultraviolet light. This type of skin has the least sebum on its surface.

## EXTERNAL BOOSTERS

Because dry skin lacks oil it is essential to remove surface dryness by using a mild exfoliator and then deeply nourish the skin by moisturising regularly to boost surface nourishment, allowing the skin flexibility and easing that stretched feeling. Sunscreen usage is vital on this skin type as it is more susceptible to the damage caused by UV light in comparison to other skin identities.

★ Oil-based cream moisturisers are best
★ Natural floral waters without alcohol are great toners
★ Rich, hydrating moisturiser used twice daily
★ Fine-grain exfoliator used twice weekly
★ Cream or no-setting masks are best for rehydration

## trade secrets

### FOR DRY SKIN

- Never use alcohol-based products on dry skin as these can make it over sensitive and even dryer!

- Use oil-based products but don't apply lots at once; thirsty skin likes gradual hydration often so apply moisturiser little but often to rehydrate the skin's surface.

- Dry skin will soak up any moisture placed on it so a good primer will provide moisture and a protective coat to make-up, preventing the disappearing foundation look!

- Anti-ageing products can be useful but never expect miracles; use products you enjoy using and can afford, otherwise your routine will become stressful and unpleasant.

- Use a rich night cream as this is the time your body rests and recuperates whilst redirecting its energy to the skin and other organs.

## DRY DELIGHTS

- ◆ Usually pores are hard to see as they are small and tight which looks great!

- ◆ A lack of sebum will make this type of skin easy to apply make-up to and it will stay on all day and well into the evening.

- ◆ No shiny patches means no spots or blemishes.

## DRY DISASTERS

- ◆ Skin can feel and look rough and dry with a distinct lack of oil.

- ◆ It can be flaky and feel taut and this type of skin is prone to fine lines and wrinkles.

- ◆ Sometimes small blemishes called 'millia' can appear around the eyes to indicate dryness. These look like very small, hard white spots which are very difficult to remove and often have to be treated professionally with a lance.

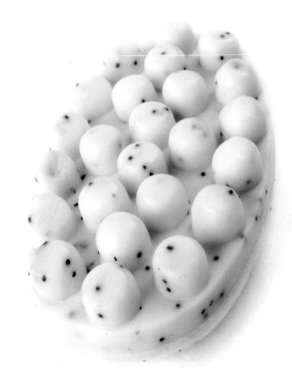

▲ Scrub away flaky skin with a fine-grain exfoliator.

# Dehydrated skin identification

Most of us have dehydrated skin caused by a lack of water both internally and externally. This is exaggerated by the effects of urban living, pollution, sun bathing and our love of fizzy drinks, coffee and pre-packaged foods which all dehydrate the body. This type of skin is identified by gently squeezing the skin together and seeing very small, silvery lines on the surface. Patches appear on the thinnest areas of the skin, such as the forehead, neck and around the eyes.

## EXTERNAL BOOSTERS

This skin needs water not oil, so all cleansing products and moisturisers should be water-based. Too much oil will just lie on the surface of the skin so when choosing make-up bases go for hydrating rather than moisturising. Dehydrated skin can prove to be delicate and slightly thinner than dry skin so when exfoliating use a liquid AHA (Alpha Hydroxy Acid) lotion for an effective but milder result. Gel products work well on this skin type as they are full of water, and sunscreen lotions are better than creams or block sticks.

★ Water-based lotion cleansers are best wiped off with cotton wool

★ Citrus waters are naturally great toners

★ Light gel or lotion moisturiser used twice daily

★ Liquid AHA exfoliator or face brush once a week

★ A gel or cream mask twice a week will rehydrate the skin's surface

## trade secrets

### FOR DEHYDRATED SKIN

• Water-based foundation products tend to dry easily so use a bit more to create the same look as a cream or lotion base.

• Dehydrated skin can crease easily so make sure the foundation base is of a medium coverage and light texture to prevent loss of moisture when the skin absorbs the water from the product.

• A regular facial spritz is the best way to feed this water-deficient skin with moisture throughout the day.

## DEHYDRATION DELIGHTS

◆ Thirsty skin normally shows little shine which helps when applying make-up as the surface is even.

◆ Dehydrated skin is not usually flaky or tight so it feels comfortable to wear.

## DEHYDRATION DISASTERS

◆ Dehydrated skin needs constant attention so regular nourishing is needed both internally and externally.

◆ Dehydrated skin identification is usually missed or overlooked, so always treat your skin for dehydration in conjunction with its normal type to save confusion and mistreatment.

◆ Fine lines and wrinkles can prematurely age this skin so ensure you protect it with SPF every day.

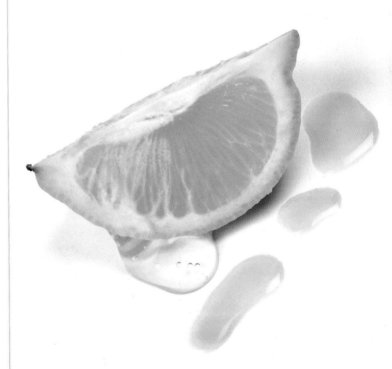

▲ Thirsty skin absorbs water fast so top up your skin regularly throughout the day with water-based products.

## Oily skin identification

Particularly common in young adults, oily skin is characterised by an all-over shiny complexion, often redness and a number of blemishes namely comedones (blackheads), pustules (whiteheads) and papules (raised red spots). Excess in sebum is found mostly on the nose, chin and forehead (the T zone), however, very oily skin can have a hypersecretion of oil all over the face and neck. In some cases acne results in younger adults but usually subsides by the early thirties at the latest.

### EXTERNAL BOOSTERS

Never try to dry out oily skin with harsh chemicals and alcohol as it will just produce more oil to return the skin to its 'normal' condition. Clean this skin type well and include toning and moisturising with a balancing water-based moisturiser in your daily routine to keep the skin soft and to remove excess oil and shine. Water-based make-up will last longer than the oil-based variety which will slide off easily. However, don't be conned into thinking powder bases are better as they can attract oily patches on the face and congeal in these areas leaving a patchy and uneven surface.

★ Water-based lotion cleansers are best removed with cotton wool

★ Tone with a citrus or lavender natural spritz

★ Apply a light gel or lotion moisturiser daily with skin treatments to prevent blemishes

★ Exfoliate using a facial brush or absorbent mask twice weekly

★ Mild clay-based fixing masks used twice weekly clear and deep cleanse pores

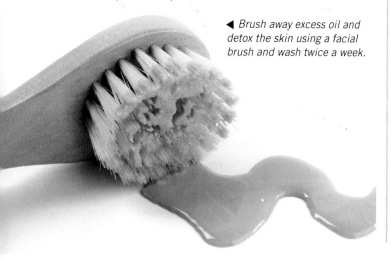

◄ *Brush away excess oil and detox the skin using a facial brush and wash twice a week.*

### OILY DELIGHTS

◆ It is found predominantly in young skin and it often remains youthful and flexible for longer.

◆ Oily skin takes much longer to show signs of ageing and will develop fewer lines and wrinkles.

◆ Oily skin remains supple for longer and has better elasticity which means that sags and bags will be fewer in this type of skin.

### OILY DISASTERS

◆ It can be very difficult to keep make-up looking even over shiny areas so a water-based foundation is essential combined with translucent powder.

◆ Oily skin tends to have open and obvious pores which can also be a make-up hindrance.

◆ Oily skin is often coupled with spots and blemishes, giving the skin an uneven texture.

## trade secrets

### FOR OILY SKIN

• Try not to cleanse an oily skin with a facial wash as often the oily surface of the skin is not cleaned properly because oily sebum and water do not mix. Use a lotion cleanser and then tone for a fresh feel.

• If sebum shows through make-up simply blot with a tissue as the moisture will be lifted from the skin but the make-up will remain as it is a heavier substance.

• Apply moisturiser all over the face, not just on non-oily areas, to achieve the perfect canvas for make-up. Matt primers are great on this skin type.

• Avoid shiny face products as oily skin is naturally shiny so don't double the effect!

# Mature skin identification

Skin begins to age rapidly from the age of 21 so we do not have much time to look young! However, we can prolong the youthful glaze to our skin by looking after it. Mature skin classically tends to be dry and shows signs of sun damage, such as pigmentation irregularities, liver spots and other mole-like blemishes. It is also identified as being lined and is nearly always dehydrated. A loss of elasticity increases sags and bags, and a slower skin immunity can reduce the protection the skin provides against bacteria and substances which cause allergic reactions. This in turn increases the sensitivity of the skin and the need for extra moisturising protection throughout the day.

### EXTERNAL BOOSTERS

Depending on internal heath and hormones as well as the environment and time of year, mature skin is normally slightly dry or dehydrated. Treat it with as much moisture as it can take and always protect this skin type with sun block. Damage has already occurred to this skin over the years so be extra vigilant and treat it carefully – harsh chemicals and perfumes will dry the surface and make it look dull so a regular spritz will go a long way to dramatically improve this skin's appearance through the day.

★ Rich creamy cleansers are best
★ Natural aromatherapy waters are great as toners for mature skin
★ Rich, regular nurturing with a treatment moisturiser, lotion or gel and sun block is essential
★ Small grain or a light AHA exfoliation is best once weekly
★ Regular creamy moistening masks help retain moisture

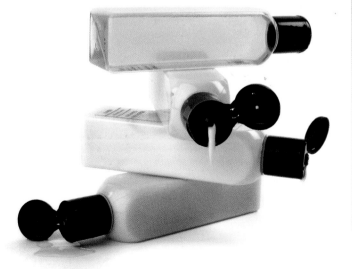

### AGEING DELIGHTS

◆ Thinning of the skin can give the illusion of a clear complexion, aiding make-up application.

◆ If you have good skin chromosomes you will always have good skin throughout your life.

### AGEING DISASTERS

◆ Fine lines and wrinkles can cause make-up application problems when products seep into the expression lines. Use cream-based products to reduce the effect of lines and wrinkles.

◆ Over years of sun exposure numerous pigmentation marks can occur. Always use sun block to prevent further sun damage but a little extra concealing work will help diminish existing blemishes.

## trade secrets

### FOR MATURE SKIN

• A cream product of any kind can prove heavy on mature skin so try gel applications around the eyes and lips to maximise absorption.

• Anti-ageing products can be very expensive and promise the earth. Be aware that the skin is an excellent barrier to outside substances. If the product is oil-based it will have a great deal of trouble getting through! Even water-based products contain very large molecules which are far too big to enter the deeper layers of the skin.

• Try to use natural aromatherapy-based products as essential oils have a very similar molecular structure to human hormones and are small enough to enter the skin and rebalance from the inside out.

# Sensitive skin identification

Sensitive skin is rare but on the increase. It appears as red, inflamed, blotchy and hot. Many people assume they have sensitive skin, however, this tends to be 'sensitised' skin as it is just the products they use which are unsuitable. Truly sensitive skin can barely be touched without a reaction. Redness alone is not a sign of sensitivity, just of a thinner or highly vascular skin. Usually this skin type is difficult to maintain and to treat. It can, however, retain a youthful appearance and vigour that other skin types lack.

## EXTERNAL BOOSTERS

Sensitive skin is often hot and flushed so cooling the skin will feel comfortable. Use a cleanser that is water-based and gentle. A cool toner with no alcohol, colour or perfume will rehydrate without causing irritation. Moisturise well and always apply sunblock to prevent further sun damage and sensitisation.

★ A light cream cleanser will soothe the skin
★ Spritz with lavender or cucumber waters
★ A light gel or lotion with a SPF of 25 is essential
★ Very rarely use a light large-grain exfoliator or facial brush
★ Cooling or creamy gel mask which does not set twice weekly
★ Cool the skin regularly with eye and skin gels to release heat and reduce flush

## trade secrets

### FOR SENSITIVE SKIN

• Do not over-treat or be harsh with this skin type as it will just rebel with a reaction which could be unsightly and set your skincare back days.

• Protect, protect, protect is the aim with sensitive skin. Look after this skin type and it will look after you!

• Always try skincare and make-up testers before you buy otherwise you may end up with a whole host of unusable products. Pick well and be comfortable.

## SENSITIVE DELIGHTS

◆ Although difficult to treat, sensitive skins are usually highly vascular which appears as a natural flush. Many people envy this brightness to the skin colour as it can appear youthful.

◆ Usually thinner, this type of skin can also appear healthy and well textured. A prime base for make-up.

## SENSITIVE DISASTERS

◆ Sensitive skin can be challenging to treat as it reacts to cosmetics and cleansers so it can be difficult to find products to suit this skin type. But products containing no alcohol, perfume, artificial colours and preservatives are on the increase and are very often more suitable.

◆ This skin is sun sensitive and can react badly so ensure a sun block is applied daily for protection against all UV light.

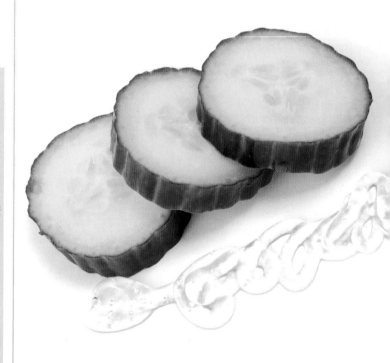

# Internal boosters

Yes, skin does need nutrients and water to look healthy and fresh but that is old news, we have known that for ages and we still crave help! Because skin is an organ like any other it also desperately needs rest, recuperation and a chance to fight the bacteria and toxins attacking it daily.

### 'SLEEP', THE SKIN SEDATIVE

At night our skin cells repair damage to the skin and heal blemishes which may have occurred during the day. Energy used for movement during the light hours is redirected to functioning organs and so the skin becomes active at night, rejuvenating and recouping for the next day. Treating the skin to a layer of nightly nourishing moisturisers can help to prevent surface dryness and lock in vital moisture. We will soon become aware if our sleep offering is too little as the lymphatic functions of the skin will show tell tale signs of neglect, like dark circles and puffiness under the eyes.

### 'LIFE', THE SKIN STRESSER

If you want to achieve perfect skin don't live to excess! Stress, alcohol, coffee, tea, air conditioning, pollution, sugar, smoke and many, many more factors surrounding us attack our skin every minute. The trick is to protect the skin rather than try to treat it! A good moisturiser will do this until you remove it at the end of the working day so invest and reap the rewards of the ultimate skin defender… moisturiser!

### 'DIET', THE SKIN INDULGENCE

Although scientifically the food we eat has little to do with how our skin looks a healthy person may well suffer less with problematic areas on their face. I recommend simply to build up the defences with antioxidant food boosts, such as vitamin- and mineral-rich fruits and vegetables as well as oil-rich fish and pure water. These may or may not make a difference to your skin but replacing these essential fatty acids and rich vitamins A, C and E will ensure that if the outside doesn't glow, the inside certainly will!

### THE BODY CLOCK

Hormones, enzymes and body cells have a huge voice in the conversation of skin. They can have a dramatic effect of what we see when looking in the mirror, and recognition of that can help us go easier on ourselves. Hormone levels can fluctuate dramatically throughout the 24 hours of the day

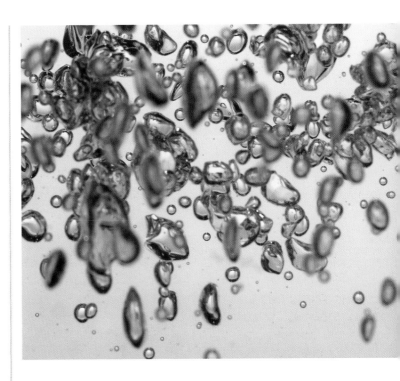

and this can lead to redness, blemishes and changes in skin texture. Stress, pregnancy and even the monthly menstruation change the balance of our hormones, with men also suffering changes in testosterone and androgen levels which have an effect on the skin.

Clearly, staying as stress-free as possible is ideal but can be unrealistic. One thing we can do to help our hormone levels and our skin is to take deep breaths wherever and whenever possible. This surge of oxygen in the system will boost the working capacity of the cells in the body and the increase in oxygen to the brain helps trigger responses to lower blood pressure and heart rate, adding a rush of nutritious oxygen to the skin and reducing adrenaline levels in the blood to slow the stress response.

## Giggling your way to gorgeous skin!

Endorphins are the body's feel good boosters. They are released when we are happy, when we exercise and when we eat foods we love. Many people use stimulants like caffeine, fizzy drinks and chocolate to boost their endorphin levels and make themselves feel happy but the best tried and tested way is to laugh. Taking the time to think of a happy or funny moment can release a surge of these happy hormones which will in turn balance your stress levels far quicker than anything else. Try it and see if these happy thoughts make a difference to your stress levels!

## Cleanse

Cleaning the skin is essential to maintain a healthy complexion, and in order to give your skin a clear chance of rejuvenating at night you must remove your make-up before bed! (If you can't, get someone else to do it – it's important!) Some of the world's top models use spring water to wash their faces twice a day and some use thousand-pound specialist cleansing creams! Whatever you use make sure it is effective and removes the surface make-up and daily dirt as well as the unseen bacteria, dust, dead skin cells and pollution.

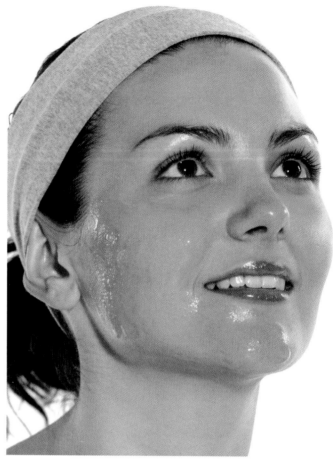

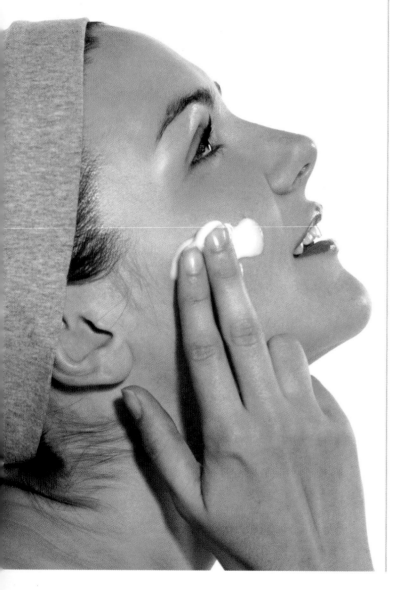

### CREAM CLEANSERS

Quite simply the best cleansers on the market, they cling furiously to make-up, mascara, dirt, pollutants and grime, and tend to be gentle on the skin's surface. These can be oil- or water-based to suit the different skin types, however, natural cleansers are best as they do not contain perfume, colours or preservatives which are responsible for 46 per cent of all cosmetic allergic reactions. Always remove make-up with a cotton pad and follow with toner to prevent an oil barrier being left on the skin.

### WASH-OFF AND GEL CLEANSERS

Water-based wash-off cleansers are not the best at removing make-up and dirt as the oil molecules in make-up do not stick to water well. However, wash-off cleansers can be good for those who wear little make-up because they freshen the skin and physiologically the user will feel toned. Younger skins tend to benefit from a wash-off cleanser as it is quick and easy, ensuring that it will be done at least!

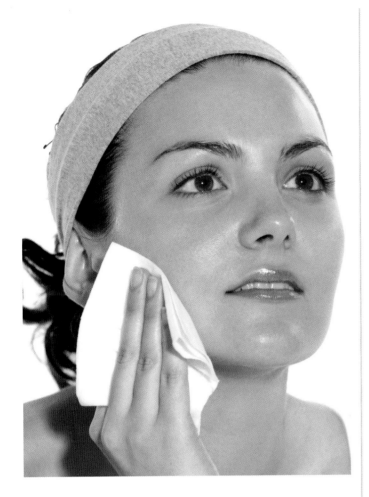

as well as pollutants and free radicals.

Soap is made of either animal or vegetable fat and caustic soda, a strong alkaline substance. During heating these products go through a process called saponification, forming salts in the soap mix. Naturally this blend of salt, fat and alkalis has a very unpleasant smell so even odourless soaps will still contain perfumes to disguise this smell.

It is the alkali in soap that makes it an ineffective cleanser because it reacts against the soft acidity of the acid mantle and destroys it, stripping the skin of its protective barrier and leaving it open to invading bacteria. That in itself is not soap's worst attribute!

Because soap is a water-soluble substance the ingredients from the soap stick to the surface of the skin, which is oily, without cleaning it a great deal. Once rinsed the residue of the soap lies on the surface of the skin and it is this that gives the after effects of feeling tight and squeaky clean.

So soap is not an efficient cleanser and it goes some way to making skin conditions worse as well as not killing very many bacteria!

### DUAL-PURPOSE PRODUCTS

Cleansers that advertise themselves as a 'cleanser and toner in one' or towels which have the same function are quick and easy to use but look closely and you will find you need to use several to get the same effect as a cream cleanser. They also contain a high level of alcohol which is why they dry out so quickly when not packaged. Alcohol dries the skin and causes sensitivity. Lotion products which also claim a dual effect turn to water in any kind of heat so be aware when carrying them as part of your make-up kit!

## The soap scandal!

As a skincare specialist I know all too well the uselessness of soap and its wash-off liquid soap friends. However, you may not be aware of the full horror that is SOAP…

The skin has a natural barrier called the 'acid mantle', a fine layer of acid that coats the skin to provide a surface uninhabitable for most bacteria. Along with sticky sebum, these make an effective barrier against nasty skin invaders

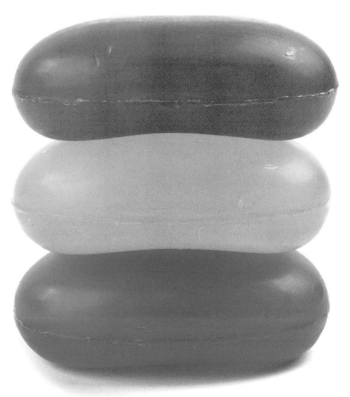

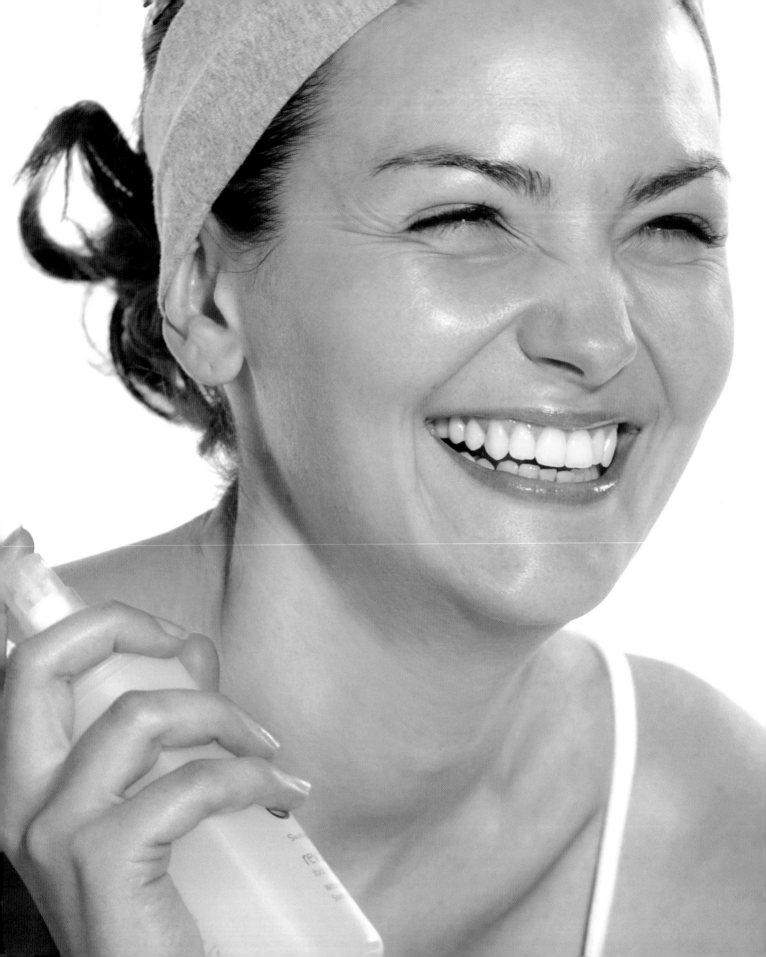

## Tone

Toning is arguably an important phase of skin cleansing. The best way to decide if you need a toner is to use it and see if you miss it when you don't. Using toner gives a psychological feeling of having clean skin, but what is it actually doing to the skin? Well, toning does have several purposes despite dermatologists arguing its usage:

★ Toning ensures the removal of all excess cleanser and surface pollutants as these are usually thick, oily substances that lie on the skin after cleansing and can cause blocked pores and blemishes.

★ It freshens the skin and cools it which helps to reduce redness and sensitisation caused by cleansing products.

★ Because the base of all toners is water, it hydrates the surface of the skin and gives it a moisturised, healthy appearance.

★ Toning provides an oil-free, clean surface to apply moisturiser to and will not block the passage of moisture into the skin as it does not act as a barrier.

There are many types of toner. The best are those which are natural floral waters as they are usually free from synthetic perfumes, alcohols and harsh preservatives which can all sensitise the skin with regular use. Spritzing over make-up can also be done during the day if the spray is fine enough as the water will evaporate without leaving lasting marks in the make-up. Toning is optional but it gives the skin a fresh, squeaky-clean feel that you wouldn't otherwise get.

## Moisturise

Moisturising all skin types is vital for two main reasons:

★ Moisturisers lock in the skin's natural moisture preventing drying and dehydration.

★ They provide a barrier to pollutants, dirt and toxins which could harm the skin or cause blemishes.

Using a moisturiser with an SPF should be standard nowadays but make sure you insist on using one with an SPF of at least 15. Remember that the skin on the face is some of the most delicate on the body and the sun is the biggest skin ager, so prevention is better than cure.

Moisturisers will be sold at a vast price range, from a few pounds to a few thousands! But as long as the product you use suits your skin you shouldn't need to break the bank. Using designer brands can be trendy but consider the basic functions you want from a moisturiser and how often you use it. Whatever you go for, you should be able to afford to buy it regularly.

Skin can change during the seasons and climate alterations will ensure your skin has different needs at different times of the year so adapt your skincare routine to mirror your skin's requirements. Many people use a heavier moisturiser in the winter and a lighter one in the summer. This change can only help your skin and introduce new ingredients which may greatly benefit it.

I would always recommend moisturising even if it is just a light gel as it provides an excellent base for make-up and it always makes the complexion feel soft, smooth and replenished. Psychological? Possibly, but feeling great is what it is all about, however you manage to do it!

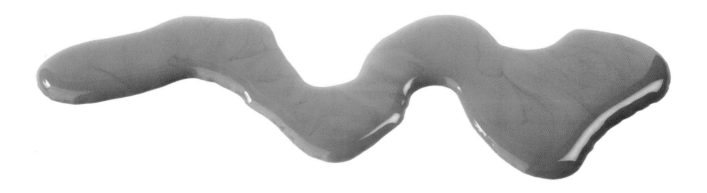

# Scrub

Exfoliation is the best way to achieve a clear complexion as it is essential for removing the dead skin cells that cling to the skin's surface. Often pollution and free radicals can stick to the skin as they are oily substances and this can lead to a dull, dirty skin. Exfoliation should therefore be a part of your regular weekly skin spa treatment. It allows make-up to lie smoothly, especially in the nooks and crannies like the nose where it is hard to remove unwanted substances.

Stimulation like this to the skin's surface is also great for increasing blood and lymphatic flow to the cells of the skin, allowing them to grow, repair and reproduce faster, giving that fresh glow we all crave. Sun damaged skin often looks dull and can get that 'leathery' appearance, making us look old before our time. Manual exfoliation will brighten the skin and gently scrub off the unwanted dull cells that give the skin this look.

**Oily skin** should be exfoliated twice a week with a fine-grain scrub. Use circular movements on the face to help clear the excess oil and reduce the risk of blemishes by boosting the immunity of the skin and helping it fight bacteria more readily.

**Dry skin** is best exfoliated once a week unless you suffer badly from flaky skin, then increase to twice a week. Use a facial brush first, then either a liquid AHA product or a fine grain scrub to really boost the skin's nutrient delivery. This will give a fresh flush to the skin, making it look and feel natural.

**Sensitive skin** may only need exfoliating once a fortnight. The trick is to use a product that will have the desired effect without over stimulating the skin and increasing its sensitivity. Try a liquid or mask preparation and cool afterwards with a moisturising gel.

**Mature skin** can be dryer and increased fine lines means that gentle is definately the way to go. Over stimulation can drag the skin and regular use may contribute to accelerated signs of ageing. Exfoliate once a week and use a gentle beaded scrub; because the spheres are completely rounded there are no jagged edges to harshly treat the skin. Alternatively, try a liquid exfoliator that can be washed off.

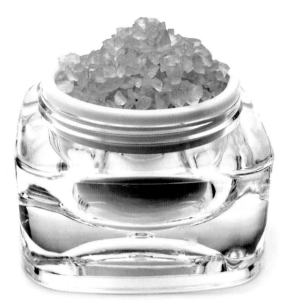

▲ Fine-grain exfoliating particals are kinder to the skin than nut, kernel or large-particle scrubs.

**Sun damaged or thickened skin** is best suited to once weekly exfoliation, but to really boost circulation ensure you massage the face first and scrub after as this will give the best result because the skin will have been pre-softened and prepared.

Never use harsh nut kernel scrubs as these contain very sharp particles and can scrape the skin unnecessarily without actually exfoliating!

## Mini skin spa

Often people try to unsuccessfully cover baggy eyes and dark circles with make-up alone. I, however, ensure all my clients have a mini lymphatic skin spa before applying make-up to try to naturally reduce problem areas before camouflaging them with make-up. A quick routine is all that is needed and can make all the difference when in front of the camera!

The aim is to stimulate the nourish centres of the face, temporarily improving the circulation of blood and lymph to the skin which will help remove toxins and boost the skin's immunity against bacteria. The facial will also brighten the skin and relax the skin around the eyes to reduce puffy eyes and drain dark circles.

The lymphatic system is responsible for removing toxins and excess water from the body. When this system is stimulated it gives the skin a paler appearance.

Blood is carried around the body in the circulatory system. Blood's main function is to distribute water and feed cells with the nutrients and oxygen needed to remain healthy and fully functional. When the blood is stimulated in the face, the skin will turn pinker, ensuring the cells in the skin get a nutrient boost.

The bones of the face help define your features. For instance we often talk about distinctive cheek and jaw bones as being attractive features. Massaging around bones feels heavenly as the muscles attached to them are slowly being relaxed. But remember to never massage directly over protruding bones as this can feel very uncomfortable indeed.

These detailed diagrams show where the vessels, bones and lymph nodes are found in the face and neck. Working over vessels and nodes stimulates the right areas to really detox and rejuvenate the skin of the face.

## FACIAL CIRCULATORY SYSTEM

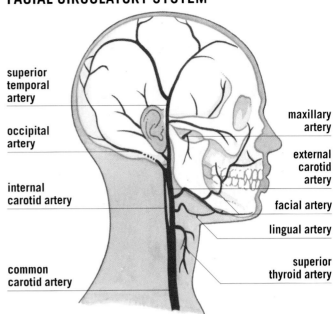

▲ Always encourage blood flow towards the heart to help stimulate a boost of oxygen and nutrients to the skin.

## LYMPH NODES OF THE FACE AND NECK

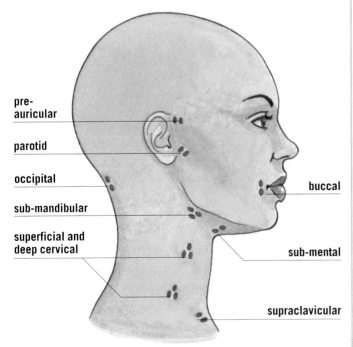

▲ By lightly massaging the skin on the face and ending each movement at the facial lymph nodes, you help to stimulate the detox zones, reducing puffiness and dark circles.

## BONES OF THE HEAD AND FACE

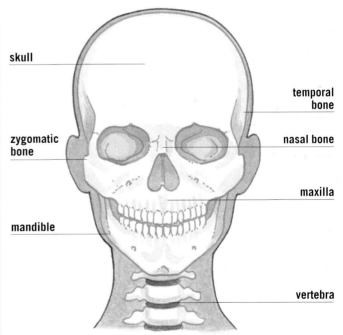

▲ Massaging lightly over bones and deeply around bones feels great as well as aiding the passage of nutrients from the blood to the bone through its surface periostium. This revitalises the skin and helps facial bones to be healthier.

# how to...

## DO A MINI SKIN SPA

Do a mini skin spa once a week to keep dark circles and sallow skin at bay! Before you start thoroughly cleanse and tone. Separate eye cleanser is not always necessary unless you have sensitive eyes, in which case use a gentle eye cleanser.

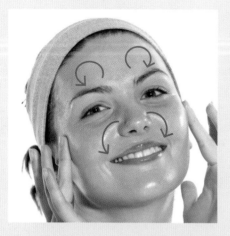

① Apply a small amount of warm facial oil or an apricot or almond oil to the skin with your fingers using gentle circular movements to distribute the oil and warm it on the skin.

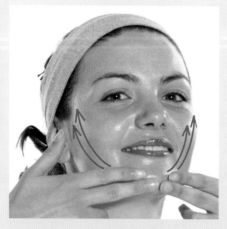

② Starting in the middle of the chin slowly and lightly slide your fingers out towards the ears. Once there, lift off the hands and repeat the movement.

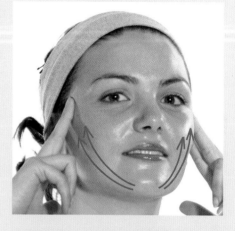

③ If done correctly the skin should appear whiter not pinker. This shows that you are moving lymph and not blood to the detox lymph zones in front of the ears.

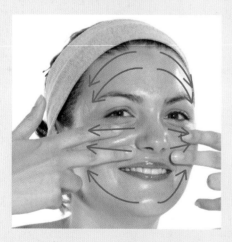

④ Using the same movement work up the face in lines allowing your facial muscles to relax as much as possible. When you come to the forehead work down towards the ears.

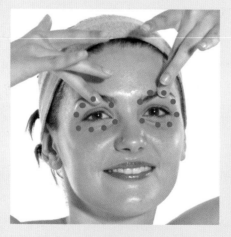

⑤ Finish every movement you make around the eyes at the lymph nodes to enable the drainage of built-up toxins. Make light, circular movements around the eyes from outside in, then gently press around the edge of the eye socket bone to help reduce dark circles.

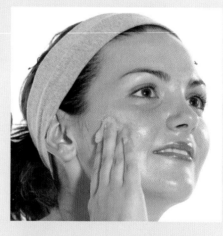

⑥ Exfoliate with a fine-grain facial scrub – the finer the grains the more polished the effect will be. Wash off the scrub and facial oil and apply a mask that complements your skin type. Finally apply moisturiser and then make-up.

## TYPES OF MASK

**Gel masks** are great for oily, congested, dehydrated and sensitive skins because they are not heavy and contain little oil whilst being cool and staying cool!

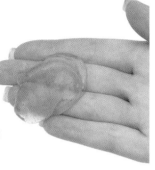

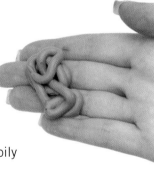

**Cream masks** are great for dry, mature and sun-damaged skin types as they contain copious amounts of oil and have a great softening effect.

**Clay masks** are ones that dry to a tight finish. These are designed to draw out impurities and deep cleanse. They can be used on all skin types but work best on oily and congested skins.

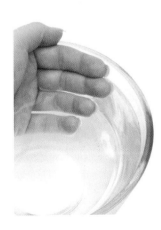

**Liquid masks** usually have an AHA ingredient that resurfaces the skin. These can be left on the face under make-up. Beware not to over treat the skin with these as you will only increase the skin's sensitivity by thinning its epidermal layers.

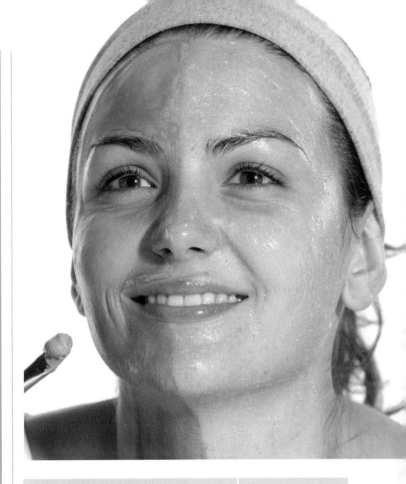

## trade secrets

### FOR SKIN TREATMENTS

- Don't overspend on night and day creams. Skin needs protecting 24 hours a day so one good SPF moisturiser will do for anytime of day.

- Avoid using eye cream directly before make-up application as it does not absorb quickly. An eye gel may be better but be sure to let either dry well before applying make-up.

- Sometimes you may develop spots or blemishes after a facial treatment because of the detoxing effect it has. Whiteheads are caused by bacteria being destroyed by white blood cells and forming pus. So squeezing spots can rid the body of this waste pus but be careful... if you squeeze too hard or too often you can damage the skin and cause permanent scarring.

# Eyebrows: nature or nurture?

Eyebrow contouring can make a big difference to a face. It changes the appearance of the eyes and face as well as making room for character-enhancing make-up.

Work around your natural eyebrow shape. Squint your eyes to detect exactly where the bulk of the eyebrow lies and tweeze around this bulk to give you the best natural shape. The arch of your eyebrow, if you have one, should be just above the outer side of the iris. This allows the eye to appear wider and deeper.

If you have straight eyebrows with no arch learn to live with them! I have and I make the most of them, as I am well aware I cannot make hair miraculously appear where it doesn't naturally grow! Whatever your eye shape always opt for a natural and tidy look as this is far more sophisticated than ultra thin and pointy!

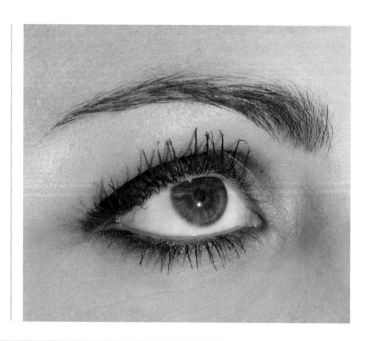

## how to...

### ASSESS YOUR EYEBROW ARCH

By following the steps below you can assess where your arch should lie and where your eyebrows should start and end for the best natural look.

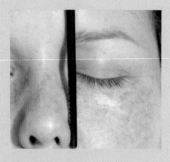 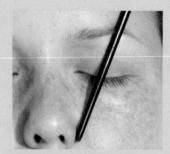 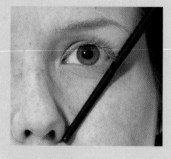 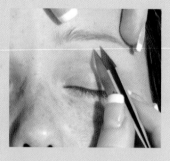

① **Align the brow brush from the side of the nose to the inner corner of the eye. This shows you where the brow should start so pluck away any hairs found on the nose side of the marker to prevent a unibrow!**

② **Angle the brow brush from the side of the nose as before and line it up with the pupil. This is where the arch should naturally appear so if the hairs are untidy here pluck away the excess to develop an arch in the brow.**

③ **To achieve the correct length to the brow, align the brow brush from the nose to the outer corner of the eye. Pluck away any hairs found on the hairline side of the brush.**

④ **Once you have a guideline to work with remove the unwanted hairs. To ease any discomfort stretch the skin with two fingers; this will open the follicle and help the hair slip out. Often an ice cube or mild numbing cream can help to reduce pain during plucking but be sure to seek medical advice should cream enter the eye.**

# how to...

## PLUCK YOUR EYEBROWS

Invest in a good pair of slant-edged tweezers for your eyebrows as this will help you create the best shape quickly and more effectively. There is nothing more annoying than grappling for the same hair several times because you have blunt tweezers that don't grip!

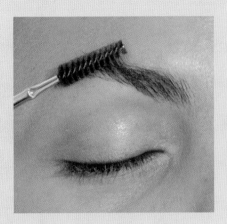

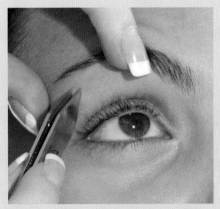

① **Start by brushing the eyebrow hairs up with a brow brush. Then measure your brow (see opposite) and using white eyeliner pencil draw over the hairs you wish to remove.**

② **Stretch the skin and pluck away unwanted hairs. Never remove more that you initially covered in white liner pencil until you have done both brows. Remove only one hair at a time and alternately pluck one brow then the next to give you a constant balance between the two.**

## FILLS AND GAPS

Never remove eyebrow hairs from the top of the brow as this lowers the appearance of the brows. Whip out any rogue hairs but do not remove more than you need to – this area is better off bleached. Should mistakes be made or hairs naturally missing, brush on some brow powder or pencil to fill the gaps. Comb for a neat finish.

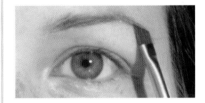

▲ *Fill in gaps with pencil or brow powder.*

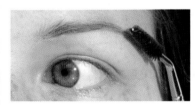

▲ *Smooth hairs with a brow brush.*

## trade secrets

### FOR EYEBROW TREATMENTS

- Don't follow fashion when it comes to eyebrow contouring; if you pluck too much the hairs may never grow back, so be warned!

- Plucking and waxing hurt so stretch the skin with your fingers where possible and always pull the hair out in the direction of growth when plucking.

- Try to pluck from the root of the hair but be careful not to be over zealous and grab a bit of skin, too!

- Always pluck the brow which is not your strongest side first; it is easy to over pluck when using the stronger hand so start on the opposite side.

- If you wax, remove the strip as quickly as you can but always stretch the skin taut at the same time. This will prevent redness, possible bruising and over drying of the skin.

- If your eyebrows are very sparse use eyebrow pencil to redefine the shape you'd like, but remember, go naturally and follow your eye socket shape otherwise you could be looking in the mirror at a clown!

# how to...

## WAX YOUR EYEBROWS

I would always recommend getting a wax from a professional! It's sticky, unpredictable and hot so please don't run the risk of 'no brow' and visit a salon! If you are feeling brave, however, here's how to do it:

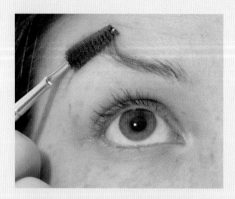 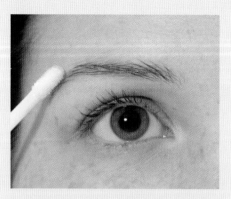 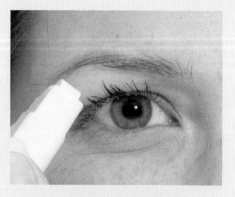

① Clean the brow and brush the hair upwards using the brow brush so all the hairs are pointing to the hairline.

② Apply petroleum jelly as a barrier on the hair you don't want removed and cut the spatula and wax strips to size.

③ Apply wax to the brow in the direction of the hair growth. Pull the strip away against the hair growth whilst stretching the skin to prevent discomfort.

## BLEACH YOUR EYEBROWS

Bleaching brows is becoming increasingly popular as people want to be in control of the colour of their brows rather than leaving it to nature. It is really easy to do and here's how.

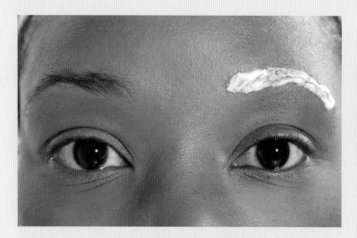 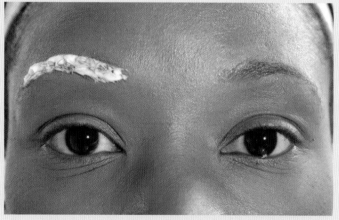

① Cleanse your brows and brush them upwards. Following the manufacturer's instruction apply the bleach to the whole eyebrow and leave for the stated amount of time. The longer the bleach is on for the lighter the brow.

② When the bleach has been rinsed off, shape the brows if necessary. If you think they are too light simply apply eyebrow pencil or tint them until you have the colour you desire. You can even go really wacky!

# Tinting and perming

Tinting and perming of lashes is a growing phenomenon and now many salons perform these lasting treatments regularly.

## TINTING LASHES

Tinting is a non-permanent process where lashes and brows are made to look darker. The effect lasts for about 4 to 6 weeks or until the hair falls out. Ideally you should go for a colour that suits your natural hair colour or skin colouring, but choosing a colour that mirrors your favourite mascara colour can give an unnatural but stunning effect, too.

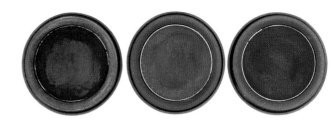

▲ *Block eyelash and eyebrow products.*

## PERMING LASHES

Using perming lotion and neutralisers, perm rods are applied to the eyelashes to give a permanent curl that lasts four to six weeks. Different rod sizes give slight, natural or exaggerated curl to the lashes so choose the size that best suits your needs. The application process is the same regardless of how much curl you want. This treatment removes the need for eyelash curlers, so crimp away!

### Straight and clean lashes

Apply perm rods and perming lotion following manufacturer's instructions. Lashes will remain curled for a number of weeks and will really help to open the eye and lengthen the lashes.

## TINT COLOURS FOR LASHES

 **Blue/black** Is ultra dramatic, the blue gives inner depth to the black and also makes the result last longer. Avoid on very fair skin.

 **Black** Suits everyone and all those who wear black mascara should use this tint. It's a fabulous look that lasts about one month.

 **Brown** A natural colour for blonde and grey hair, it can appear very dark to begin with but over the first few days will diminish to a natural colour.

 **Grey** A very light finish only really used on older clients or those particularly worried about tinting. The results will be fine for a first timer but very fair.

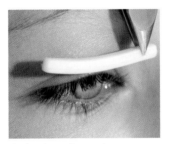

▲ *Apply curling rods.*

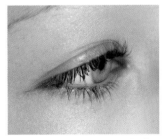

▲ *The end result is stunning!*

## trade secrets

### FOR TINTING LASHES

- If the tint goes in your eyes it may sting but don't panic! A few blinks and a bit of water later and you will be just fine.

- No, you can't make your lashes lighter! So don't even try!

## trade secrets

### FOR PERMING LASHES

- Do not open your eyes as the permanent lotion can be a strong irritant!

- If you have straight eyelashes that are not sticking well to the rod, use some lash adhesive to stick them around the rod; they can be tamed!

- Always follow manufacturer's instructions as products differ dramatically and you want the result to be the best it can.

## EYELASH EXTENSIONS

It is very popular to extend lashes and this can be done in one of three ways:

**Individual lashes** are best used on the upper outer side of the eye to exaggerate the length and width of the eye. Trim them if they are too long before applying the glue and use tweezers, not fingers, to position them on the root of the hairs.

**Strip lashes** give a voluptuous thickening effect and can be very dramatic. Pre-cut if necessary and use glue and tweezers to avoid sticky fingers!

**Eyelash growth** enhancing products can be expensive and usually contain collagen and elastin to moisturise the lashes and help them appear longer and in better condition. The effects will only last as long as the hair is in the follicle so regular use is essential.

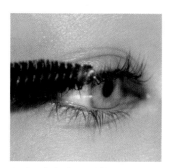

▲ *Apply lash conditioning treatment every day.*

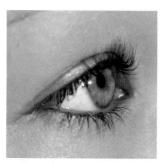

▲ *Conditioned lashes can appear thicker.*

## trade secrets

### FOR EYELASH EXTENSIONS

- Use lash glue sparingly and avoid getting it in the eye!

- Use tweezers to apply lashes as fingers will adhere to the glue and it can end up being a messy process.

- Don't pull false lashes off as more often than not natural lashes will be stuck to them and you will be left with a bald patch! Instead use a proper glue dissolver for gentle painless removal.

# Facial waxing

Facial hair can be a hindrance so many people like to wax the upper lip or facial region on a regular basis to avoid foundation and powder congealing in the hairs.

### DOS AND DON'TS

Waxing is easy to do but also easy to get wrong. Here are a few do's and dont's.

### DO:

✔ Clean the skin thoroughly before waxing as wax will stick to make-up and produce a slippery surface so the hairs will not be removed properly.

✔ Apply the wax thinly. Too much wax will make it hard to remove and you could end up in a sticky situation!

✔ Remove the wax quickly and stretch the skin to prevent redness. Apply an after-wax lotion to cool the skin immediately and if red heat bumps appear apply a cold compress for 10 minutes to reduce their appearance.

### DON'T:

✘ Overheat the wax as this will burn the skin and you'll still have to remove the wax with the strips which can be painful.

✘ Don't use moisturiser on the area for about eight hours as it contains perfume and alcohol, which can exacerbate redness and cause an allergic reaction.

✘ Don't overwax the area. If any hairs remain after the first attempt try to pluck them out instead as the skin will be stressed. Make sure you only wax the hairy bits as overwaxing could encourage more hairs to grow which is not the aim of the game!

✘ Never wax over broken or irritated skin. Wax removes dead surface cells and will make any skin condition worse.

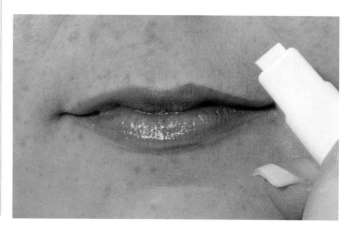

# Chemical boosters

Peels are commonly used by cosmetic surgeons and dermatologists to resurface the skin on the face, neck and hands, essentially burning away the surface layers of the epidermis to eliminate fine lines, scar tissue and signs of sun damage and pigmentation. The deeper the peel the longer the recovery – from one hour to months.

## FOR A GRADUAL RE-SURFACING OF THE SKIN

Light peels like AHA (Alpha Hydroxy Acids) are milder and are used mainly as exfoliators but a higher strength can have a clearing effect on pigmentation and uneven skin as it works to remove the first layer of the epidermis. Microdermabrasion is similar in its effects and strength but utilises sharp sand-like particles which are powerfully applied to the face and sucked off to reveal this deeper exfoliation effect.

## FOR ANTI-AGEING AND REMOVAL OF WRINKLES, FINE LINES, SCARS AND PIGMENTATION

Medium strength chemical peels which use trichloroacetic acid are more wearing and can reach the dermis of the skin easily. They require a recovery time of around three weeks and skin will show signs of healing by becoming initially very red and developing a crust scab which will flake of in a week. These types of peel are very uncomfortable and most practitioners advise a course of pain relief whilst in recovery. The total healing process takes weeks and pigmentation in the skin can be disturbed.

## FOR A DRAMATIC TREATMENT TO ELIMINATE SCARS, TATTOOS AND ACNE PITS

Deep layer skin peels like phenol are very strong and remove the epidermis and most of the dermis leaving a very swollen, scab-encrusted, painful result for a number of weeks. It is so strong that often your natural skin colour will be paler after a peel and will never revert back to normal. You are also warned very strongly never to allow the sun on your 'new' face and will be expected to wear a mask bandage over the face for at least eight days. This is a serious operation and is very painful so being treated by a doctor is essential. Dermabrasion has similar results but is gruesomely performed, as high speed sanding or metal brushes are used to 'scrape' away the epidermis and virtually all the dermis. Recovery times can take months with a complete healing time of six months.

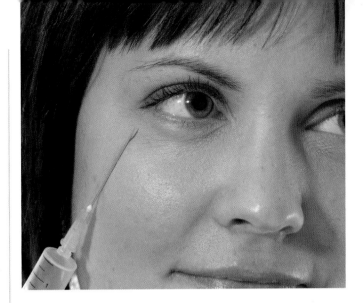

Many people are choosing to regain a youthful complexion with the help of Botox, collagen injections and creams. Topical creams have a temporary effect if at all as the skin is a very effective barrier and it will be almost impossible to get collagen ingredients into the dermis of the skin where it is found naturally. Injected products will be far more effective and will last from eight weeks to six months.

## BOTOX

Botox is a cosmetic form of the toxin 'botulinum'. It temporarily blocks the nerve impulses from the nervous system to the muscles, causing the latter to freeze. Used on areas that show expression like the eyes and forehead, lines and wrinkles are reduced but expression is difficult. In Hollywood, celebrities have been extending the uses of Botox to prevent sweating under the arms and to ensure their high heels do not tire their feet by having injections in the soles of the feet!

## COLLAGEN AND FAT TRANSFERS

Collagen injections have been used for many years to plump out wrinkled areas and add volume to lips. The appearance is temporary and does not prevent wrinkles. However, to avoid the infamous 'trout pout', where lips have been oversized either due to too much treatment or an allergic reaction to the collagen, always be treated by a professional. Bovine collagen is used from specifically reared cattle and there is a real risk of allergic reactions so patch tests are vital! Fat transfers are common in those wishing to harvest their own fat cells for the plump look, however, in areas of expression it does not last as long as other similar treatments and the recovery time is longer.

# Sunscreen

Every time we step outside the sun's rays shine on our skin and generate a reaction that causes the skin to produce melanin, turning our skin brown. Melanin is our only natural defence to the sun, so additional protection is needed.

## UVL

Ultra-violet light is given off by the sun even when it isn't sunny! This light is divided into three types UVA, UVB and UVC. The sun has been proven to be the worst cause of skin ageing and as we now know causes skin cancers. It is also responsible for skin pigmentation, growths and mole changes.

★ **UVA** This type of ray is not filtered by glass, it will penetrate to the deeper layers of the skin, easily damaging the skin from within. Unlike UVB, UVA light is constant and can damage regardless of how bright the sun is shining.

★ **UVB** Is more superficial and is therefore usually responsible for sunburn. UVB does not penetrate glass and is at its strongest when the sun is high and bright during the hours of 10 am and 2 pm.

★ **UVC** This type of ray is normally completely absorbed by the ozone layer but it is thought that with damage to the ozone layer more UVC skin damage will be seen in the coming years.

The sun causes collagen in the skin to break down and become less effective. This reaction encourages the production of elastin fibres called 'solar scars' that deform the dermis and produce lines and furrows on the surface of the skin. These manifest themselves as fine lines and wrinkles.

Free radicals are unstable oxygen molecules that also cause skin damage and diminish collagen. These are found all around us and can change the essential make-up of a human cell and warp its genes leading to cancerous cells.

When we burn in the sun our body protects itself by killing damaged cells in the skin. This manifests itself as skin peeling and is the body's way of trying to prevent serious skin damage.

Using sunscreen of a minimum SPF of 15 will protect the majority of skins on a daily basis. If you do want to tan start with a high SPF and very gradually reduce the factor. Remember, if you burn your tan will not be as long lasting

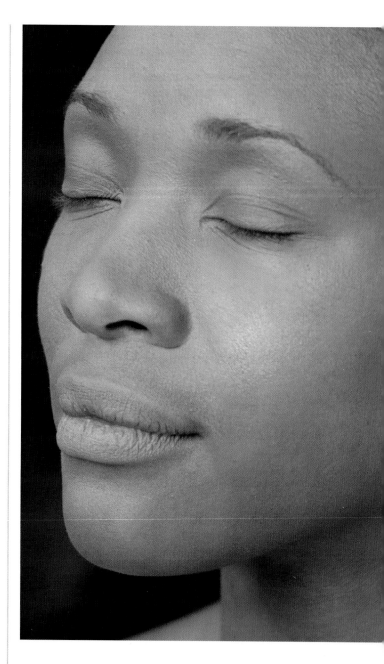

because you will peel and the tan will go with the shed skin!

Some sunscreens absorb the sun's rays whereas the better ones block the sun's rays altogether. Don't make the mistake of thinking that if you are fair you can still tan, it'll only take a bit longer! Not the case, you may just become more freckly instead!

The safest way to tan is by faking it – nothing works better for giving colour whilst staying safe.

## Make-up in the sun

As your body warms, your skin will naturally perspire to cool the body's core temperature and prevent overheating. Modern make-up will usually withstand this, however, the trick to keeping make-up on is to blot away excess water, not wipe it off.

Many make-up preparations melt in high temperatures which is why keeping cosmetics in the fridge isn't such a bad idea. However, when on holiday wear as little as possible on your face to avoid discomfort and looking like a melting waxwork! Even nail varnish can melt in the sun so going barely bare is the best plan for a fresher look in the summer heat.

## Tanning without the sun

This is safer than tanning in the sun and with the developments of suntanning sprays and slow-build body tanning lotions the chances of that streaky effect are greatly diminished.

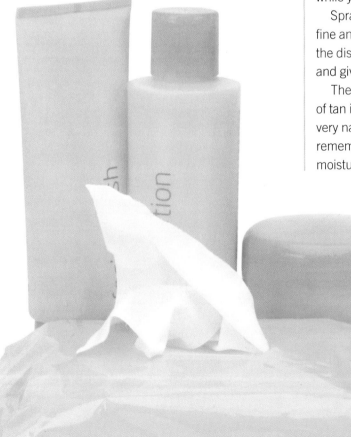

When applying self-tan mousse ensure you wear gloves and apply evenly. Mousses tend to be fine products so you may need more to achieve the look you want.

Lotions tend to streak because of their oil content so the trick is to apply a thin layer and reapply if necessary. There is nothing more boring than doing the zombie walk for hours while you dry so make a little go a long way!

Spray tan tends to dry the quickest. Pick a spray which is fine and follow the manufacturer's guidelines with regard to the distance you spray from the body otherwise it could run and give you a dripping look.

The latest tanning products are moisturisers with a hint of tan in them. These are great for a slow-build tan and look very natural. Apply thinly as they take a while to dry, and remember, because they are moisturisers you needn't moisturise your skin before applying.

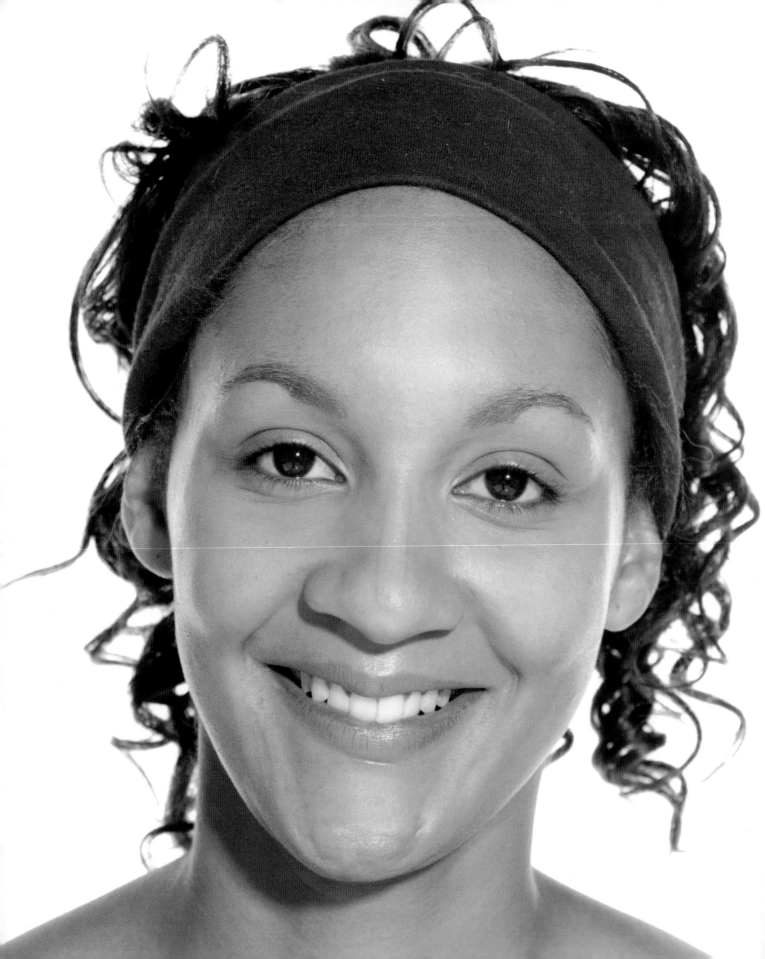

# 04 the natural canvas

# the natural canvas

It would be impossible to photograph every skin tone for this chapter because there are hundreds! So I have grouped colour types together but you are very individual and the secret to good foundation is to try one that is invisible against your skin colour!

> **You are not a 'colour' because of your ethnicity, you are just a colour, and this is what we work to complement**

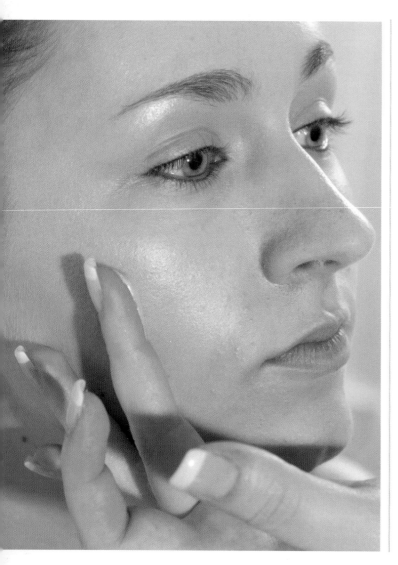

There is no doubt that in past years women with darker skin tones have been seriously undervalued in the make-up market with very little choice of colours and textures available. However, with inspiration from models like Iman and Naomi Campbell the selection has been evened out so all women and men are able to make choices freely with make-up.

The wonderful plethora of cosmetics and make-up we see in department stores should not be seen as daunting but as a sea of wonderful choice and experimentation. Often the easiest way to work round cosmetic counters that interest you in a store is to ask them why they are different. If you like what you hear delve into a selection of testers and samples. Usually the only reason samples are not given out is because they want you to feel pressured into buying there and then! Don't… Take your time and you will find the better companies will give you free samples or allow you to have your make-up done to show you what will suit you from their ranges. This will enable you to make an informed choice without wasted expense.

## Colour therapy

So what suits you? Colour is studied as a form of therapy and there are a few guidelines you may or may not wish to investigate as a bit of fun! I have known colour therapy to work wonders for inner and outer wellbeing and make a huge difference to individuals. Let's look at how we can invite colour into our lives and shatter the boundaries of our old favourite browns!

## Pale skins

If like me you are used to always looking for foundations called nude, cherub or porcelain, then this very wonderfully pale complexion matches yours. This light skin tone can be seen in redheads, brunettes and blondes with a variety of eye colours so it is difficult to come up with a set of hard and fast rules. Your base tone is the one you naturally hold without a tan but it is essential to match your foundation with your skin colour throughout its seasonal changes.

Usually this skin colour is synonymous with a fine texture, which can appear to have bluish undertones. History's make-up icons were desperate to achieve the very lightest of this look and many were unsuccessful. This skin tone does not tend to tan easily and will burn with over exposure to the sun. It can sometimes appear red but is not necessarily sensitive. Many colours look fabulous with this skin colour but owners tend to safely stick to browns, greys, black and plums. Both natural and unnatural looks can easily be achieved. The only crime here would be not to experiment with this skin tone!

### BASE COLOURS

Skin colour changes remarkably throughout the year and this range of lighter skin tones experiences noticeable change. Some skins will tan even though the base is fair, while others won't, but this tone is very susceptible to freckles and mole pigmentation growths from long-term sun exposure. Emotion is also not well hidden with this skin colour as flush shows easily, as does inner ill health in the form of dark, puffy eye circles and a grey, drawn appearance.

▲ *This range of colours varies from creams to pinks, peaches and light beige and vanillas.*

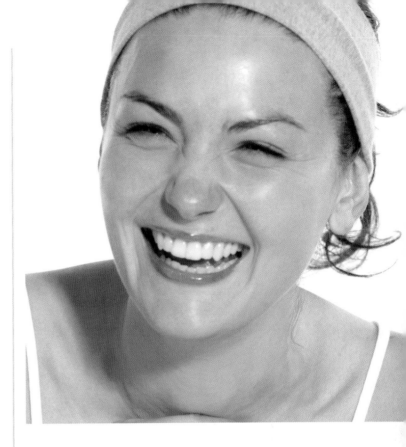

### THE COLOUR WHEEL

Blush should mirror flush! So choose either pinky or peachy tones for this skin colouring. Bronzers do look good but don't apply too much as this can make the skin look drawn. Eyeshadows are there to experiment with but browns, oranges and safe pinks can be used alongside blues, greens and very deep plums and navy.

As a rule if you want to make your eyes stand out, then reduce the lip colour. On the other hand, if you want to make a feature of your mouth, go natural on the eyes but use stronger colour on the lips. For everyday make-up, wear beige, pinks, browns and reds.

For lips, eyes and cheeks, neutral shades like browns, oranges, pinks and pastels look best on pale skin. However, although the colour choice may not be vivid don't be afraid to go dark!

▲ *Olive skin has a yellow base and so a variety of shades with a yellow, light brown or tanned base works well.*

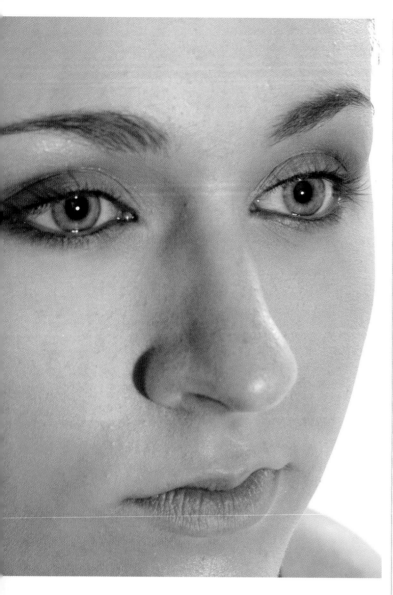

## Olive skins

These tones are rich, warm colours. Yellow tones can be added to this section, however, olive skin is easily described as such in make-up adverts and marketing tools.

A wide range of colours is welcome here and this is the one skin tone where colour is readily found. Both bright and natural colours work on this skin which can look equally sultry and awe inspiring!

Olive skin can often be a great light reflector and highlighter with less sun damage issues than its paler counterpart as this skin type has a good base of melanin to protect from unwelcome UVA and UVB rays. In general its warm, muted tones work well with most colours. Brunettes are usually owners of this skin tone.

### BASE COLOURS

Olive skin comes in many shades but as it ages it reacts in a similar way. This skin usually tans easily and rarely burns. If sunburn does occur, it often changes to brown very quickly with few repercussions. This range of skin colour normally shows ill health by turning paler, and a jaundiced sallow tinge can appear if rundown or tired.

### THE COLOUR WHEEL

Apricot and pink blushers look great on this skin tone as they bring added warmth and brightness to skin which may not have a great deal of natural flush.

Eyeshadow colours vary hugely but use smoky greys and blues, along with vanilla, greens and even violet.

For lips, reds, oranges, browns and soft pinks are really flattering and often shimmer gloss and bronze work well in the summer.

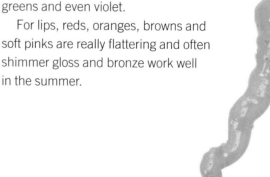

# Mocha and chocolate skins

Deeper skin tones show colour brilliantly and although there are so many lighter and darker shades in this group the colour choices are universal and flexible. It doesn't always have to be brown and beige!

Dark coloured skin tends to be shiny in appearance but is rarely oily. This shine can easily be covered but keeping a natural appearance means allowing some of the shine through and actually accentuating it with bronzer.

Darker skin tones do well in the sun, as although they do not have more melanin granules in the dermis, these do tend to be larger which helps protect this skin from the ravages of the sun and ageing. Often this beautiful array of mocha tones can be susceptible to hyper pigmentation, which is where the dermis has been damaged and has deepened or lightened in colour. This can be covered easily but it is something to be borne in mind when concealing.

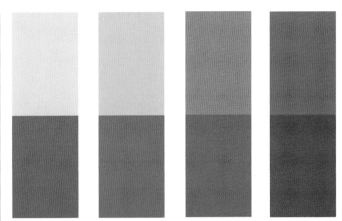

▲ Chocolates, coffee, toffee and mocha – all these delicious shades are classic black skin tones.

## BASE COLOURS

Darker skin tones can appear ashen if using products with mica in them so be aware of this when you make your choices. This skin tends to stay blemish-free and often has only texture irregularities which can be resolved with good skincare. These tones also allow the skin to look younger for longer. But protection with an SPF is still very much needed and skin damage from the sun will show as pigmentation irregularities.

## THE COLOUR WHEEL

**Blush** A deep bronzer looks great on this colour of skin and gives a slight sheen which looks sexy. Russet colours work too, and orange, rose, burgundy and gold are all stunning.

Vibrant eyeshadows can look fabulous but for a more classic look copper, browns, chocolate, chestnut and vanilla are great as well as purples, violet and bronze.

Gold, bronze, deep purple and red are nice lipstick choices but cinnamon, coffee and a simple gloss look stunning.

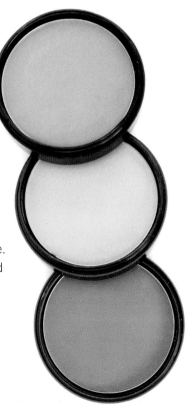

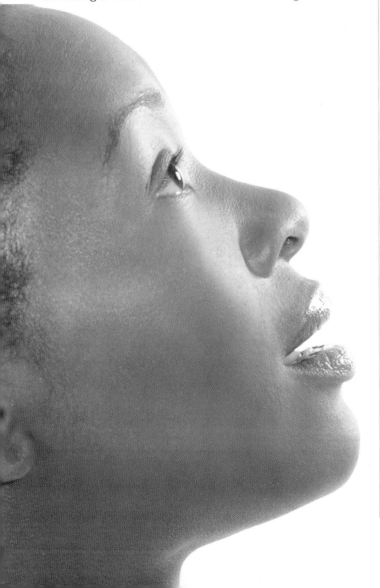

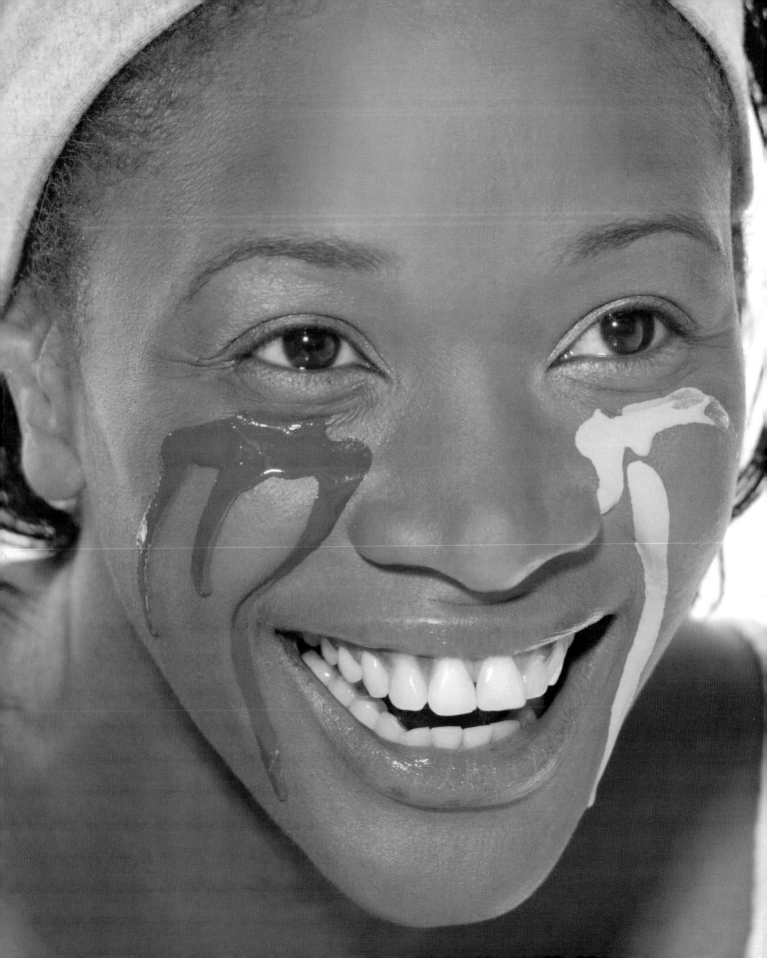

05 foundations

# foundations

Todays foundations are not just colour correctors but sun protectors, anti-ageing cosmetics and skin therapy treatments. We are in the ultra-modern era of make-up where perfection can be created, and complementing natural skin tones, colours and features should be an expected standard.

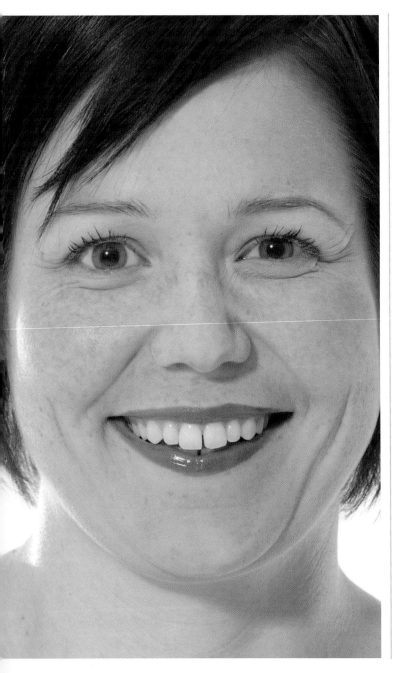

Choose a product that treats your skin identity and suits your colour. You can have both so try before you buy and insist on a tester to see the end result. Better make-up companies want to provide the best foundation for you so let them experiment and come up with one which is suitable. Always try the product on your jaw line and face, not the back of your hand! And if you can, test the base on the darkest and lightest areas on your face at the same time. This will challenge any formulation to 'blend' with your skin colour naturally.

**Skin comforter bases** These contain vitamins and SPFs to nurture and protect the skin, preventing premature ageing by fighting free radicals and treating your skin to luxury, to keep it glowing and soft.

**Light diffuser bases** These clever products work on reflecting light on the face rather than absorbing it which draws attention away from the problem areas and gives an overall even-textured appearance.

**Sheer bases** These leave a velvety finish to the skin and can look fabulous, but remember imperfections can be highlighted. This type of foundation is best used on smooth, young skin.

## Texturise

Different formulations of foundation will have different coverage and effects; try them all on your skin and see what suits you best. In the summer you will probably wish to create a lighter, more radiant look than in the winter so change your formulation, not your colour. Foundation will not give you the tan you always wanted, just a line reminding you it wasn't the right choice! If you want to increase glow, try self tan first.

## Take your time with foundation and be sure to choose the best colour and texture of base for you

### TINTED BASE

A tinted base can be worn by all skin types but is best used on those who need very little coverage. Often it provides an SPF and is spectacular used on holiday when you may just want a hint of colour but essentially a 'barely there' effect. It is best applied with fingers as a sponge will absorb too much product which can be an expensive waste.

### MOUSSE BASE

A very light and quick drying application. Most mousses are light in coverage and have similar properties to tinted moisturisers. They probably won't contains an SPF and are best applied with fingers as the sponge will absorb too much. Great for young skins and those of you who don't always wear foundation.

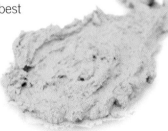

### LIQUID BASE

This is usually either a water- or oil-based liquid and is very good for dry, dehydrated and combination skins. Medium coverage will be provided and it is best applied with a wedge sponge to create an even texture. Some firmer textured liquids work well when slightly warmed by the fingers in the palm first. Experimentation will tell you the best option for your liquid's consistency.

### CREAM BASE

A medium to heavy coverage for all skin types used especially when trying to achieve a flawless complexion for photo shoots and film. This foundation will last throughout the day. Apply with fingers to manipulate the texture and lighten the application around the eyes to prevent exaggerated lines and wrinkles as the base settles. For everyday wear, only those with dry skin should use a cream base as it can be over-nourishing.

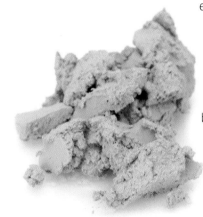

### COMPACT BASE

Easy to carry, compact foundations are normally applied with a sponge and are best on young, combination, dehydrated skins. Extremes of dry and oily skins can suffer from a lack of consistent coverage with this type of foundation as the powder will cling to dryness and slide off oily areas. I prefer using these without added water even though this is the recommendation, as they can become clogged and troublesome to apply.

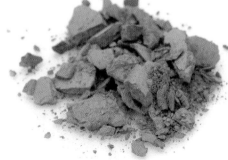

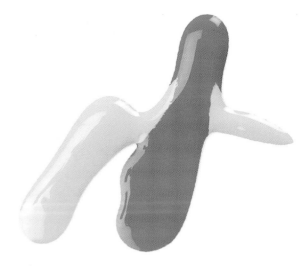

## POWDER BASE

These are different from compacts because they are almost pure powder and should really only be used to top up foundation with a matt finish or on mature skins for a light cover foundation. These can be applied with the sponge provided or a brush depending on your preference.

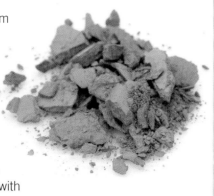

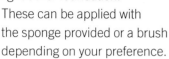

### LONG-LASTING LIQUID BASE

Long-lasting foundations are used for heavy coverage and will dry quickly so there is little time to blend these products. Practice makes perfect, however, and once on the base will stick like glue! Remember that to make this product look good you must apply and blend quickly. Often a little moisturiser added to the base before application will allow you more time to blend this product.

## CAKE BASE

This foundation is very thick for a heavy coverage. Apply with fingers to smooth the waxy base. This foundation can be used on all skin types, especially those wishing a flawless, but unnatural, base for photographs. It is very similar in texture to concealer and is just as heavy, however, used for the right occasion or on selected areas of the face it can create a terrific look.

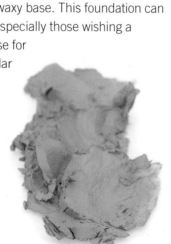

## Back to the future

The future of foundations lies with the more advanced cosmetics companies developing some amazing products, including pigmented foundations that have colour particles suspended in gel formulations to give an unbelievably natural appearance which will last as long as you wear it. Optical technology is advancing new products too, with photo-reflective liquids that contain many layers of pigments preventing the light or eye from concentrating on one area, giving the illusion of flawless skin. These pigments also allow the foundation to change colour in different lights so you will look as glowing in natural light as you would in the evening or on a photographic set!

It is astounding the amount of money and time spent on improving our complexions, especially on base and foundation products. Women of all ages are now looking and feeling better than ever and this extra confidence doesn't just come from eye or lip make-up, but from the knowledge that their skin looks glowing and healthy!

## Shading

Getting the right colour is the most important aspect of buying a new base or foundation. Try testing three colours: one which you think would be right, then one a shade lighter and one a shade darker. The best choice will be the colour you can't see. Some cosmetics companies will blend your own individual foundation at a reasonable price. This is really worth the investments as we all come in many shades, not just one of four or five set colours!

Never assume you are in a particular colour group because of your ethnic background; you may not be the same colour as anyone else in the world so never make do with the nearest colour!

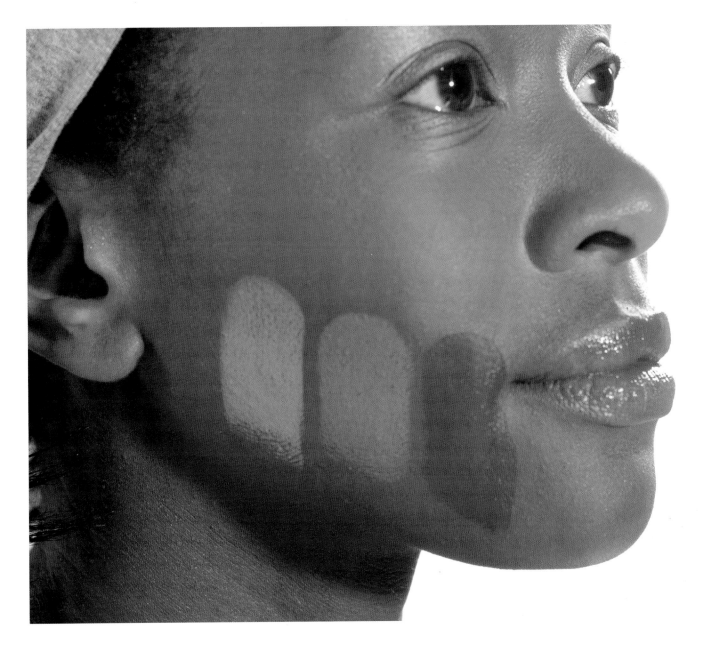

Most base foundations come in a variety of colours but they all tend to be either:

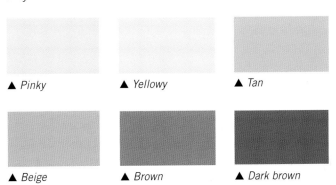

▲ *Pinky*     ▲ *Yellowy*     ▲ *Tan*

▲ *Beige*     ▲ *Brown*     ▲ *Dark brown*

To choose the right one for you look at your skin without make-up on and try to identify which of the colours on the left your natural skin looks most like. Once you pick out the nearest match, then try to find a base with this colour to achieve the best coverage.

The skin's acid mantle can change the appearance of cheaper foundations so checking your base shade will prevent any unsightly shade changes through the day. Always test foundation in natural light as this gives the truest representation possible and always colour test foundation on the jaw line to ensure a perfect match.

# Primers

Primers have been used for many years to mattify and neutralise areas such as lips and eyes before applying make-up. Make-up artists prime most areas of the face now especially if they are working under heated lamps or in air conditioned environments as these changes in temperature greatly affect the skin and the application of make-up. Even eyebrows are not past an application of primer, but a gel base is best as cream will stick and clog the hairs even if it is transparent.

### EYE PRIMER

The great thing about eye primer is that it almost totally stops eyeshadow moving during the day, which means a more lasting result to eye make-up. Eye primer is applied all over the eye lid up to the brow and so gives the perfect canvas to all make-up, including eyeliner and all shadow textures,

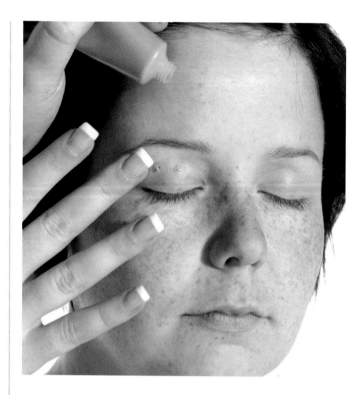

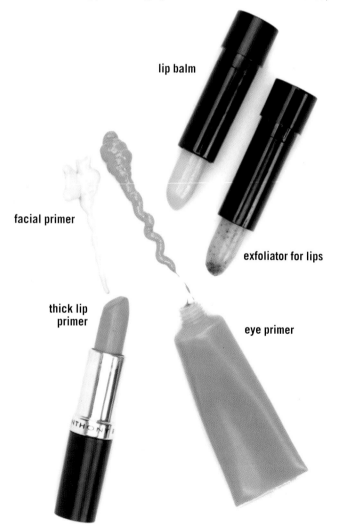

lip balm

facial primer

exfoliator for lips

thick lip primer

eye primer

especially cream shadows. Primer often allows for better blending, too, as the skin is matt and allows for easier brush movements.

### LIP PRIMER

This tube of brilliance enables anyone to achieve a completely matt finish to their lips before lip liner is applied. Lip primer is applied all over the lips and just over the edge of the lip line eliminating the risk of lipstick bleeding into surrounding skin as well as increasing the lipstick's staying power. Often gloss can destroy the appearance of lip colour as it gives the ultimate shine but the added oil encourages even the best application of lip colour to smear and run. Primer blocks this reaction and the little extra time it takes to apply can add hours to the lasting effects of your lipstick.

### FACIAL PRIMER

This little miracle is just the treatment for anyone with different textured or pigmented skin. Usually of a cream consistency, it is applied before make-up with fingers and dries instantly for a matt finish over moisturiser. Blend your foundation over the top of this base and see the difference in blending ability and the way colour lies on the skin – the canvas is far more even and easy to contour. Primer also allows foundation to last longer so on a hot night out this is a must!

# how to...

## APPLY FOUNDATION

A proper application of foundation is the make or break of good make-up. It should be smooth, even and blended well into the hairline and neck. Make sure you cleanse, tone and moisturise the skin thoroughly before applying foundation.

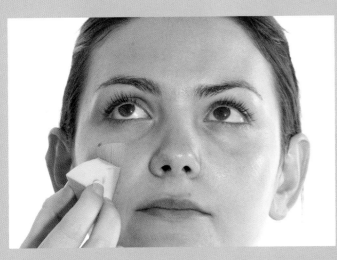

① Tinted moisturisers, cream, cake and mousse foundations are best applied with your fingers to smooth the distribution of these products. Powder, compact, liquid and long-lasting foundations are best applied with a sponge as these will need manipulating without the extra heat from your fingertips.

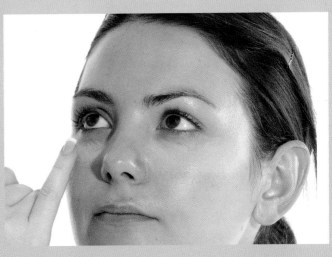

② Gradually build up coverage until you are satisfied, covering any dark areas under the eyes and around the nose area with a slightly lighter shade of concealer.

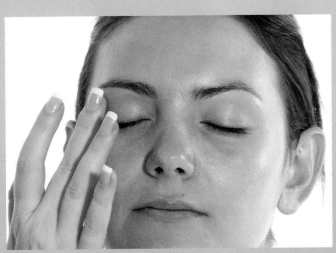

③ Work round the face in towards the T zone. Often this area will require a little more coverage so leave this until last and build up extra product if necessary. Always cover the eyelids and lips with primer as this helps provide an excellent base for eyeshadow and lipstick.

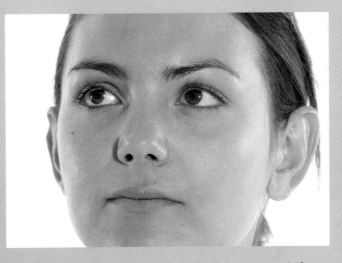

④ The end result should blend invisibly with your neck, jaw line and hairline. If it doesn't, just keep working on it until you get the result you want. If the foundation goes streaky or thick, add a little moisturiser to the face and begin blending again.

## Concealer

Surprisingly, most skin coloured concealers work best when they are applied over foundation. Because they are wax-based they need to be warm when applied to the skin and if spread too thinly will be ineffective.

Light-reflective peachy and yellow toned concealers are best for covering uneven pigmentation. Concealers that match your skin tone or slightly darker concealers are best for spots and freckles. Always choose a concealer that is one shade lighter than your skin tone when covering darker areas like under the eyes as this will help draw attention away from problem areas.

## Colour correctors

These coloured products are used to even out colour on the face. Often this cannot be achieved by foundation base alone.

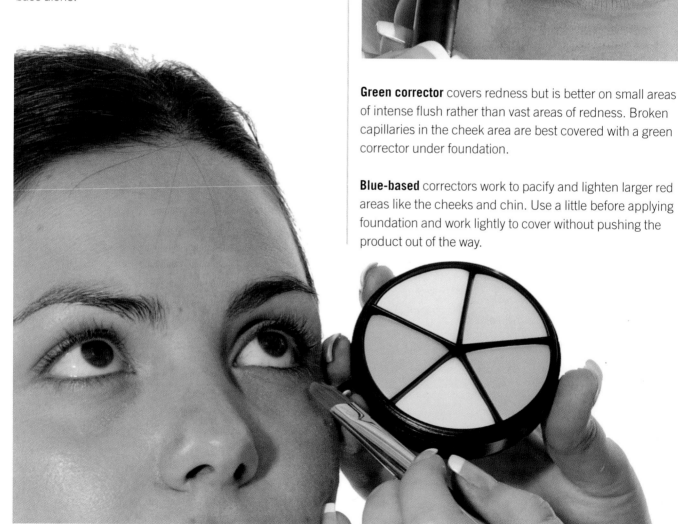

**Green corrector** covers redness but is better on small areas of intense flush rather than vast areas of redness. Broken capillaries in the cheek area are best covered with a green corrector under foundation.

**Blue-based** correctors work to pacify and lighten larger red areas like the cheeks and chin. Use a little before applying foundation and work lightly to cover without pushing the product out of the way.

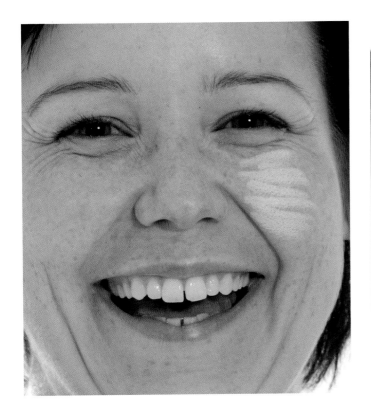

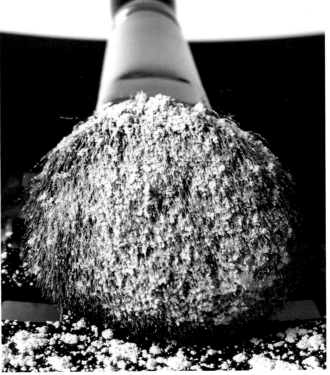

**White correctors** brighten and lighten dull skins with a lack of even colour. Use under foundation to level uneven, dull skin. Light concealers are also great for lifting dark eye circles and reducing tired looking eyes.

**Purple** contrasts yellow or sallow skin types adding a brightness and glow to these skin colours. Apply under foundation to even out unruly patches of pigmentation.

## COSMETICS UNMASKED

Foundation and concealer products contain 'buffers'. These are ingredients that prevent colour change in your foundation during the day. The acids secreted by our skin can change colour pigments but these strong buffers prevent this occurring in most modern foundations. Waxes, oils and emulsifiers blend to create the base of all types of foundation, they are just blended in different quantities. Most cosmetics firms add vitamins, perfumes and specialised ingredients to help market their products. However, if an allergic reaction occurs, it may well be the preservative in the product so try a more natural base.

## trade secrets

### COVER UP

- Colour correct the areas you need to cover, then apply foundation to the face. Use concealer under the eyes, around the nostrils and on the chin.

- Never use concealer haphazardly as a white patch under the eyes is even more unsightly than a dark circle!

- Make-up sponges come in various shapes and sizes but the classic wedge allows you to get into the nooks and crannies that others don't.

- A fine tipped brush is great for covering blemishes and patchy skin as you have ultimate precision at your fingertips.

# how to...

## APPLY CONCEALER

Concealers come in sticks, pump action pens, pallets, liquids and brush application. Often the most convenient and hygienic are the pen distributors but work with the coverage you desire, not the packaging, however much you may wish to buy the pretty one!

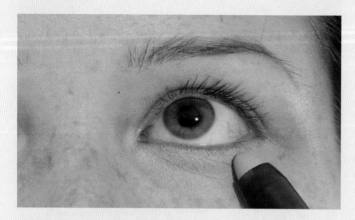

① Apply a light coloured concealer under the eye just below the problem area. This lifts the perception of the discolouration and will blend up with your foundation to cover naturally without running into expression lines and wrinkles.

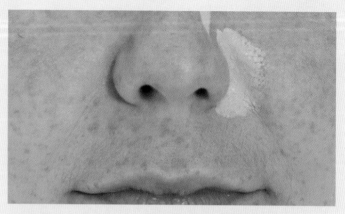

② Use a brush to apply a light-reflecting product to the nose area to diminish darkness and broken capillaries. Often your fingers are useful to help blend or thin waxy substances in the product for easier application.

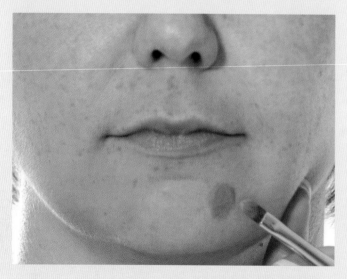

③ Choose a slightly darker concealer for blemishes as the redness will shine through regular foundation. A brush or cotton tip will be useful to apply this and if necessary blend with your finger. Apply foundation over the top for extra coverage. Try a concealer with tea tree or silic acid to help treat the spot as well as covering it.

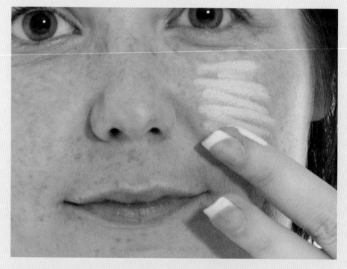

④ A little green cover applied with the fingers is useful here to cover the slight redness. Follow with a natural colour for the foundation, possibly a shade lighter, to brighten the area and draw attention away from the redness.

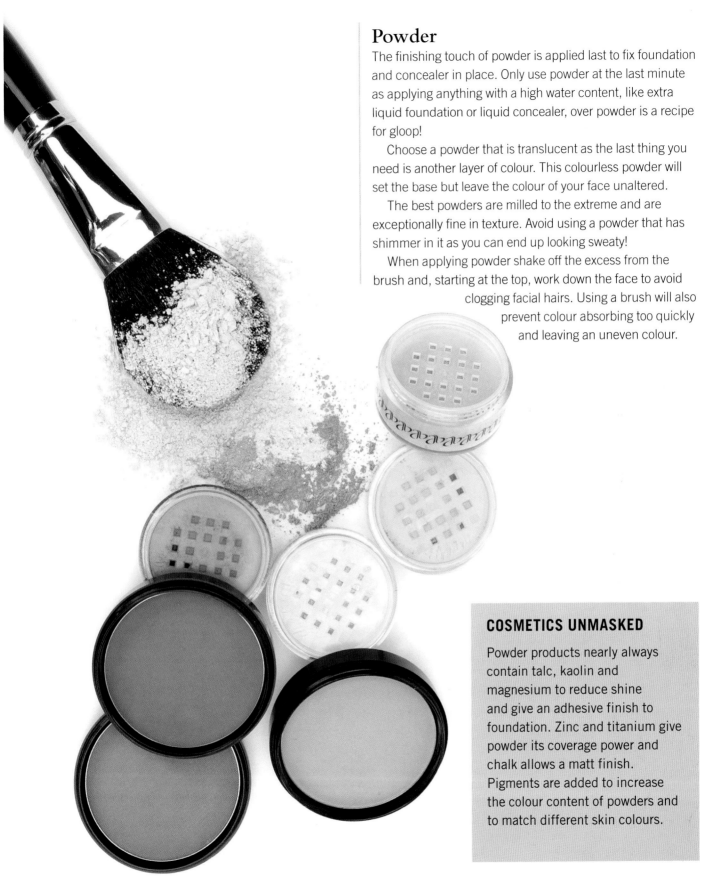

## Powder

The finishing touch of powder is applied last to fix foundation and concealer in place. Only use powder at the last minute as applying anything with a high water content, like extra liquid foundation or liquid concealer, over powder is a recipe for gloop!

Choose a powder that is translucent as the last thing you need is another layer of colour. This colourless powder will set the base but leave the colour of your face unaltered.

The best powders are milled to the extreme and are exceptionally fine in texture. Avoid using a powder that has shimmer in it as you can end up looking sweaty!

When applying powder shake off the excess from the brush and, starting at the top, work down the face to avoid clogging facial hairs. Using a brush will also prevent colour absorbing too quickly and leaving an uneven colour.

### COSMETICS UNMASKED

Powder products nearly always contain talc, kaolin and magnesium to reduce shine and give an adhesive finish to foundation. Zinc and titanium give powder its coverage power and chalk allows a matt finish. Pigments are added to increase the colour content of powders and to match different skin colours.

## Facial contouring

There is always something about our face we wish we could change. A nose that is a bit crooked or one too many chins! There is a way you can increase and decrease the appearance of your features using foundations and concealers. Celebrities are known to increase their cleavage using make-up and create a more prominent jaw line or cheek bone area. To highlight, use a lighter colour concealer or powder and to shade use a slightly darker shade than your natural skin tone.

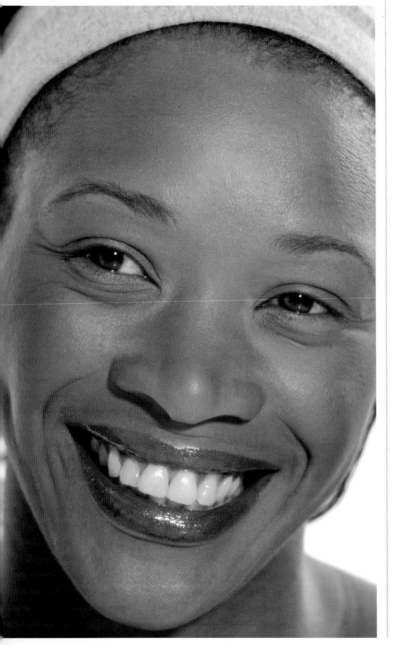

## Basic face shape contouring

We are all born with a basic face shape that is determined by our bone structure, however, it is nice to be able to distract the eye from certain parts of the face. Facial contouring to alter face shape is the application of shading and highlighting colours to do just that, by encouraging the face to appear oval, which is the most flattering face shape.

### CORRECTING FACE SHAPE WITH CONTOURING

Remember, when you want to accentuate an area, highlight it in a paler colour; if you want to tuck it away or make it appear deeper set then shade it! Always start with minimal product – the key to facial contouring is to be subtle and blend, blend, blend so that you create the effect of contouring without it being too obvious.

**Square face** Characterised as being a solid jaw line with unnoticeable cheek bones, this square face shape is contoured by adding a little shade to either side of the jaw, breaking up its solid and flat appearance. Shading the outside upper forehead also reduces the obviousness of the area. To create a more defined cheek bone area highlight above the cheek bone and apply blusher underneath. This lifts and accentuates the area of bone missing in a square face.

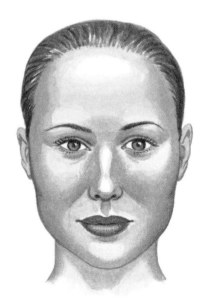

**Long face** A long face offers few features on which to use make-up so to create them shade along the hairline and jaw line to reduce the length of the face. Then highlight and blush the upper cheek bone area, being careful not to extend too far into the hairline or too far down the face.

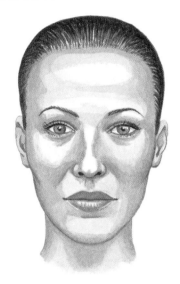

**Oval face** This is the face shape most make-up artists try to mirror! This shape offers just the right amount of structure and angularity to really apply make-up well and gain the most from your look.

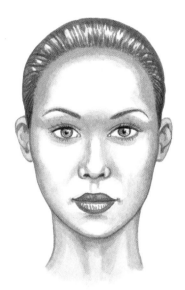

**Heart-shaped face** This face shape tends to have too much forehead width, so to reduce the appearance shade with a darker concealer or foundation on the sides of the face just above the eyebrows. Also shade the tip of the chin as this can appear pointy and shading will have a softening effect. Highlight above the cheek bones and shade underneath. On some heart-shaped faces blusher applied on the apple of the cheeks can look very natural whilst again reducing the width of the face.

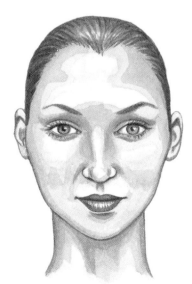

**Round face** With this face shape the cheeks are often plump and hide the cheek bones. This takes away all the natural angles of the face, so to reintroduce these simply shade under the cheek bones and blush under the cheeks, too, whilst applying highlighter to the high cheek area to create a false bone structure. Highlighting the tip of the chin can also help give a more angular point to the chin.

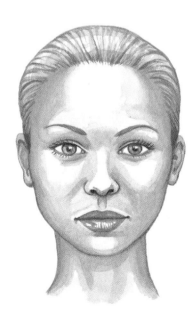

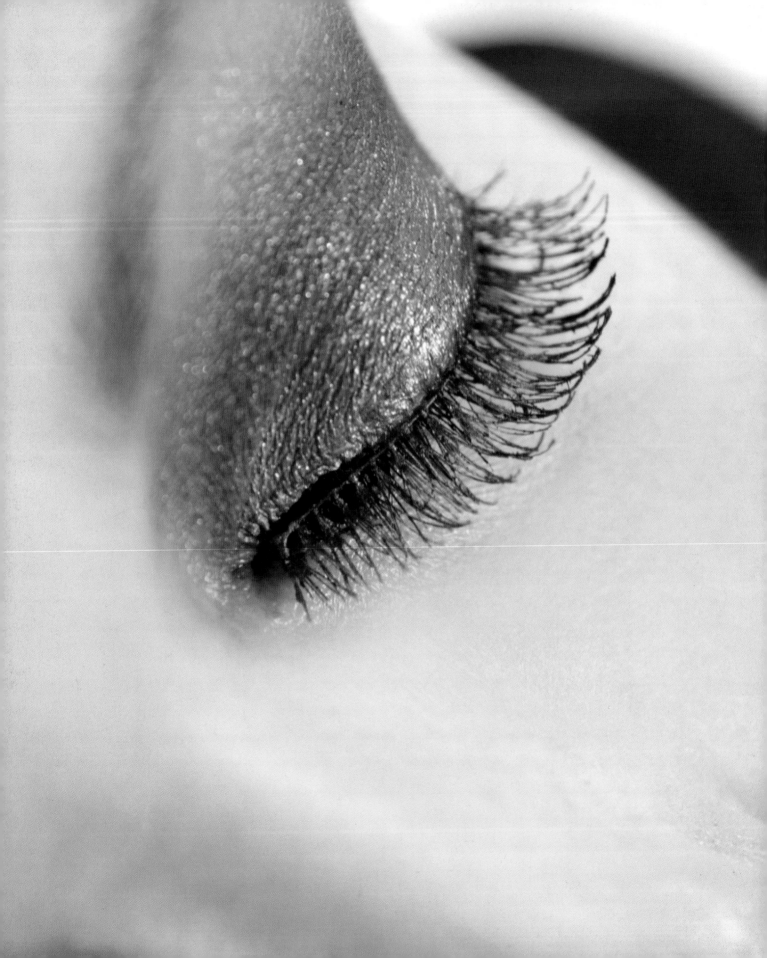

# 06 eyes

# eyes

Eye make-up can be the hardest to master but the most rewarding. The vital first impression is made on the eyes as they are the windows to the soul. Make-up fashions can dictate what you should be wearing but more often than not it is best to go with what feels right for your eyes. Once you have played around with what suits you, becoming more adventurous will come naturally, but if you love your own style then wear it with pride and glamour!

A good base to work from is essential and following a few eye reviving guidelines can help reduce puffiness and discolouration as well as brightening the eyes making them look fresh and restored.

## Bright eyes

Cucumber and cold tea bags are well known eye soothers – not because of their ingredients but simply because they are cool! The skin surrounding the eyes is ten times thinner than anywhere else on the face and so ageing and dryness affect this area the most. Cool products give a fresh relaxed feeling to eyes and psychologically wake you up.

Eye gels or eye packs and masks can also have the same effect but added ingredients such as lavender, ginseng and green tea will also superficially treat the delicate skin around the eye having a boosting effect that revives and opens the eye. Eye cooling products are also great for draining and reducing puffiness or tiredness around the eyes.

## Drainage

Lymph is a substance lying under the skin and is responsible for the removal of waste such as toxins, bacteria and free radicals from the body. To stimulate the drainage of these toxins which can cause dark circles and puffiness simply add a few movements to your facial routine that circle the eyes and end at the ear lobe where there is a node that speeds up the discharge of toxins from the body (see page 48).

## Eye eye!

It is easy to make your eyes look brighter and bigger without the use of make-up. And you don't have to go to the extreme

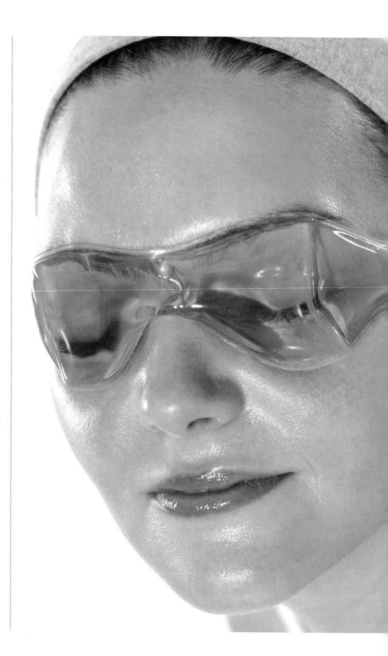

of tattooing on semi-permanent eye make-up! There are ways to accentuate your eyes temporarily that can be done regularly and because they do not affect your appearance unnaturally you will look just as gorgeous with or without make-up! The best way to perform these eye opening treatments is to follow the step-by-step guide on pages 50–54.

**Eyebrow shaping**  The creation of an arch will give the impression of a lifted eye which appears wider and longer. Simply plucking away excess hair from below the natural brow will really tidy the eye area.

**Individual or strip eyelash extensions** make a huge difference to a face, especially when applied to the outside upper lashes, adding depth, width and length to small or round eyes.

**Perming or curling** the lashes opens up the eyes and allows you to reveal more of the iris which always looks great and increases colour on the face.

**Tinting lashes and brows** gives depth to the eye area, making a huge difference to the overall appearance of the eyes without the need for make-up. It creates the impression of wearing mascara without actually wearing it.

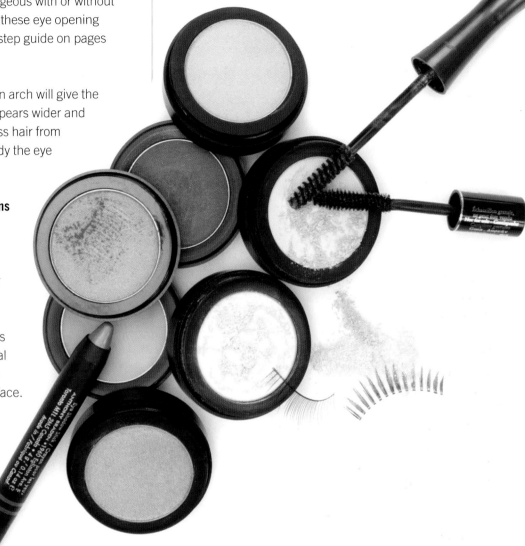

**Botox** aids the reduction of wrinkles and expression lines around the eyes. So although you may well look younger, the paralysed muscles around the eyes will not be able to show expression. Expression is a form of visible emotion so be aware that too much use of these products can eradicate the natural beauty of your emotion.

## Texturise

Eyeshadows come in many wonderful shades and textures and have been developed by cosmetics companies to battle the application problems found in the past. Blending can be a problem but with the right tools and products, it is easily mastered. Regardless of your age or eye shape try as many formulations as you can, as often more than one works but the different looks they create will help you decide on which ones to use for specific occasions.

## POWDER EYESHADOWS

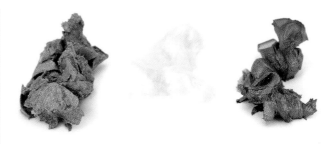

These tend to come in either matt or glittery formulas. Matt will suit all eyes but be aware that shimmer accentuates the eyes so mature or lined eyes may find this overpowering.

Powder shadows are usually the easiest to apply and the best blenders. Modern day shadows are manufactured in huge air dryers where the particles of colour are bashed around for hours with air particles and become extremely fine and dust-like. These are the best to use as the colour is intense and applies like silk. Naturally you will need less powder when the colour intensity is higher and this lowers the risk of colour lining the creases of the lid throughout the day.

Powder colours can be very dramatic but start with a pale shade and add colour and depth to the eye gradually using a sable brush. Applying powder shadow under the eye will look great for that sultry, smoky evening look. Use a little and smudge to get a terrific look. And don't worry: this can feel messy but it will look great.

### CREAM AND GEL EYESHADOWS

These are easy to apply but can be sticky and messy in hot weather. Blending is also difficult if not done with a brush. Never apply too much as cream or gel products seep into the lines on the eyelid making them look old before their time!

Cream highlighters are often the best as they contain shimmer and glitz to really reflect light and open an area of darkness, such as under the brow hairs. Remember that cream and gel products create a softer and younger appearance and will subtly enhance glow.

Cream eyeshadows can look sheer and natural, too, and often make-up for a wedding is shown best in this base. Cream shadow is best applied with a brush little by little, especially when using dark colours. Often a larger brush is best for lighter colours as it will deposit colour all over the lid much faster. A good tip if you need to blend cream shadow is to dip the brush in a little translucent powder as this enables you to blend without adding unwanted extra colour!

Gel eyeshadows are best used on their own and only on younger eyes. There will usually be little colour but a great shiny finish which is virtually impossible with any other type of shadow product.

## Pencil shadows

If they are soft enough pencil shadows can offer great definition to upper and lower lids. These blend well and often require no extra blending tools so are great for a work make-up bag.

Pencil shadows are the definitive precision tool for shadow definition. They are really best utilised in small areas for a darker or lighter line. Even what seem like garish colours look fantastic in small quantities so experiment with a pencil and then see if you are brave enough to use it all over the lids!

Colour looks best on a pale canvas so use a powder shadow as a base and then use pencil shadows to build

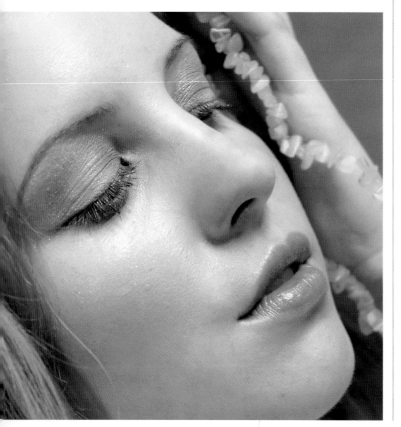

definition and shape to the eyes. Using these under the lower lids and inside the lid lines can also look beautifully dramatic.

With any eyeshadow consistency colour can seep into the creases of the lid during the day. If this happens use a brush to blend again and be sure not to apply too much product as this will slow the blending process.

## Eye correctives

Altering the shape of your eyes can completely change your look so identifying your eye shape can help open up more colour and shade options. Try to complement your eye shape by being subtle in your changes as a dramatic change may look too obvious. Remove your make-up and identify which eye shape you have.

## HOW TO CORRECT YOUR EYE SHAPE

**Deep set eyes** are those with a larger socket. Enhance the appearance of these eyes by applying a light colour over the socket and a colour (not too dark) in the socket blending up to the brow line. A liquid liner on the top lid looks great if extended slightly on the outer corner, along with lashings of mascara to top and bottom lashes.

**Small eyes** are exaggerated by applying greys and browns on the socket of the eyes and dusting eyeshadow under lower lids, too. White on the rim of the lower lid will enlarge the pupils and highlighter under the outer brow will deepen the eyes. This is easy applied and even contact lens wearers will be able to comfortably apply pencil here.

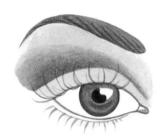 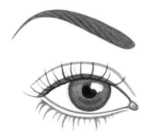     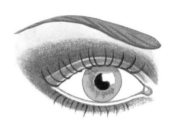 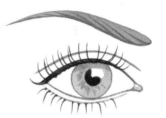

**Round eyes** need to be given length so apply a colour to the lid area only and blend up and out towards the outside tip of the brow. Highlight the outer edge of the eyebrow with a paler shadow. Apply eyeliner to the top of the lids only and exaggerate the line past the lid. Mascara on the top lashes looks great with just a light coverage on the bottom lashes.

**Long eyes** look beautiful when the brow is arched and light shadow applied up to the brow. Use a darker colour to line the socket only and blend upwards. Highlight the lashes by applying mascara to top and bottom lashes and an eyeliner pencil on the lower lid which finishes exactly where the corner of the eye ends.

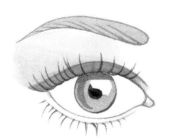 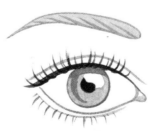     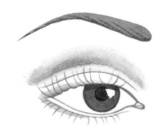 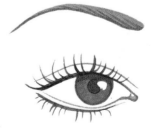

# Colour

Choosing colours can be a trial but going with a set of colours that suit your skin tone will always complement your features. These days most eyeshadows are sold in twos and threes so you instantly have colours that go well together.

**Fair skin** always looks most natural in brown, beige, green, peach and cream colours but equally can suit reds and plums.

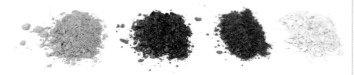

**Olive skin** looks great with most colours because there is warmth in the skin tone to counterbalance bright colours. For a natural look copper, gold, oranges, cream, purples, reds, bronze and chocolates work really well.

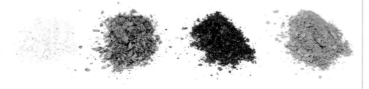

**Buttermilk and toffee skins** can look divine in a selection of vibrant colours but for a more natural look try pinks, peaches, hazelnut, plum, grey, creams and gold.

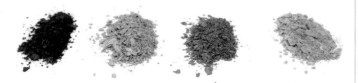

**Chocolate and coffee coloured skins** can really hold strong colours like purples, reds, navy, bronze, gold, black and grey but again for a natural finish try ivory, copper, bronze, oranges and browns.

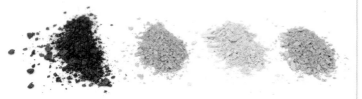

# Eyeliner

Eyeliner has been used for thousands of years. Even Cleopatra made her eyes appear larger using a wisp of colour around the eyes. In India children are shown how to use eyeliner at a very young age as it frames the face and instantly enhances any look.

### EYE PENCILS

A good eye pencil is a great investment. It should be soft and easy to apply; the worst pencils are ones you have to rub on as these make the eyes water and sensitises them. Greys, browns and plum are best for fair to olive skin but if you want to make a statement go for black every time.

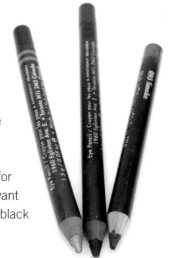

### LIQUID LINERS

Liquid liners come in many forms, from fine brushes to blocks of solid colour. For the sake of hygiene, some make-up artists use block liners as they are easy to sanitise. Both work well to create that imposing dark line which gives maximum impact day or night.

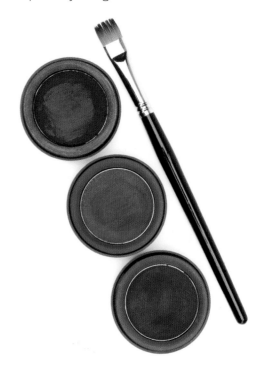

## APPLY PENCIL LINER

A soft pencil is the best and most dramatic tool to enlarge the eye area and it can be manipulated to create a cream shadow effect or a solid black line. Choose your desired look and perfect your technique.

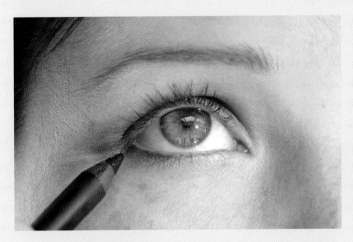

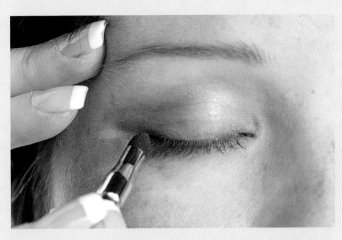

① Apply pencil eyeliner by stretching the eyes to smooth out any lines that could hinder the smooth line application. Don't panic if you get the shakes; blending this line will smooth out any wobbles.

② Using a sponge blender, smudge the liner out towards the edge of the eyes. If you like the look of liner inside the eyes then apply to the rims of both the top and bottom lids for an ultra sultry look! Be aware that this will shrink the eyes' overall appearance so if you have small or round eyes this inner lid line may not complement your natural eye shape.

## APPLY LIQUID LINER

Liquid liner is the naughty girls' liner! It is tricky to apply but once on it has the most powerful effect of all your evening make-up. Liquid liners come in many colours but often the original black is the best choice.

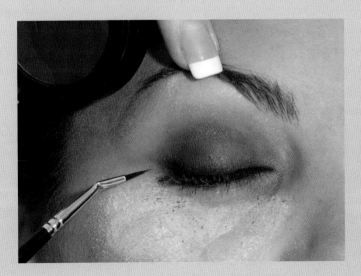

① Stretch the eye lightly to eliminate wrinkles and lines. The best way to finish the line is to relax the eye and with a steady hand apply a second coat to the lids. Liquid liner always looks best on the top lids. If your hand shakes under pressure start either with a pencil line and work over the top with a liquid liner or simply do a series of dots on the lid and blend together to join them.

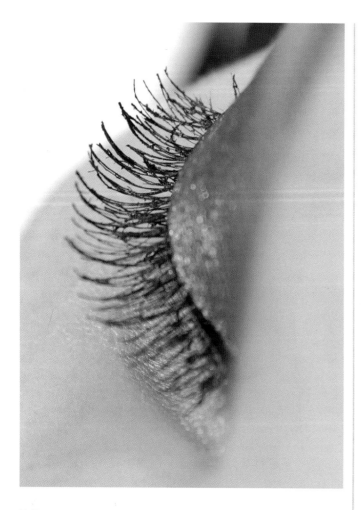

## Mascara

This is my sister's favourite make-up product and one she wears unbelievably thick, but it looks great! Not the chosen style for everyone but mascara's diversity can be really amazing!

Light feather lashes that are long and dark usually only appear on men or camels! So often we need to create this desired look with the help of mascara and false lashes.

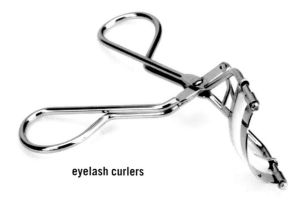

**eyelash curlers**

### COSMETICS UNMASKED

Liquid mascaras are usually water-based which means they can easily be removed. Beeswax reinforced with nylon fibres helps lengthen the lashes. Polymers and resins prevent smudging and make the product waterproof. Vegetable oil allows mascara to be applied easily and coats the lashes to condition them and prevent the product drying out.

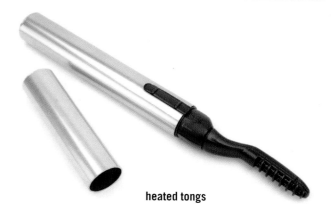

**heated tongs**

Mascara always looks better on curly lashes so using curlers or heated tongs first will enhance the lashes' appearance.

Use curlers on clean lashes and pump the curlers lightly when they are on the base of the lashes for about 15 seconds. This allows for the ultimate curl to develop. Remember to release your grip before pulling away otherwise your precious lashes will be pulled out! Heated curlers can be useful but tend not to give as much curl definition.

If this look is enough for you just set the lashes with a clear mascara. If volume is what you want, then use mascara to add length and breadth to lashes.

### LUSH LASH

Modern day mascaras contain silicone to extend natural lash length, however, you can buy extension treatments such as fibres and white lengthening products which help build a luscious length. The look is outstanding but be careful with these products as they can make lashes brittle over a number of hours and break off leaving you with shorter eyelashes and a crumbly face!

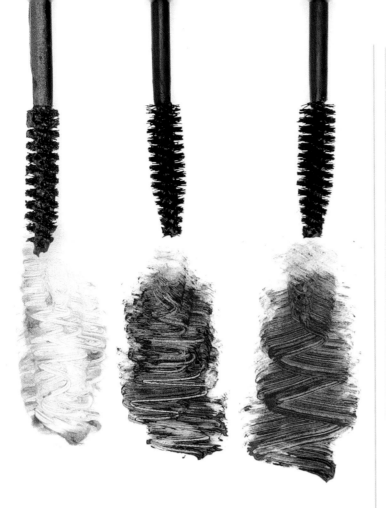

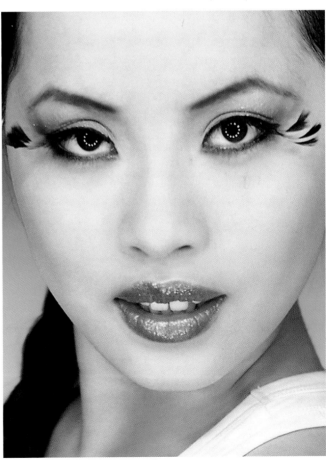

## trade secrets

### FOR MASCARA USE

- Don't blink when applying mascara; you are increasing the chance of splodges.

- Avoid quick movements when applying mascara as this encourages lashes to stick together. Take your time and apply it slowly, and you will find the definition much better.

- Remove blobs of mascara with a lash comb and a cotton bud for splashes.

- Try not to sneeze whilst applying mascara as the results are interesting!

- Avoid pumping the brush inside the mascara tube too much as this traps air in the product and dries it out.

Apply mascara in thin layers to get a feathery appearance. Use a colour that complements your eyes and a wand that adds volume to your lashes.

Creeping back into modern make-up, cake mascara can create an excellent look but it will be heavy and can be unhygienic. Nowadays we use water to dampen the block but saliva was used in the 1960s!

If you have very fair hair, then this heavy look will be strong and dramatic but if this is the look you desire, then cake mascara is the only product for you!

## Falsifying evidence!

Lash extensions come in many shapes and sizes and traditional black has been added to with bright colours, silvers and even flowers! For a natural look, curl your lashes and apply individual or strip lashes to the base of your lids with glue. For a more vampy look try something different like feather lashes and lots of bright eyeshadow!

# how to...

## CREATE DAY EYES

For everyday wear eyes can be subtle and natural whilst still being stunning. A variety of colours can be used but matching shadows with your clothes and accessories will complement your whole look.

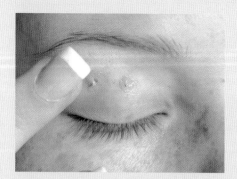

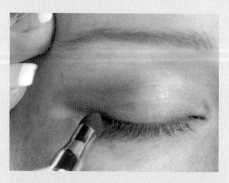

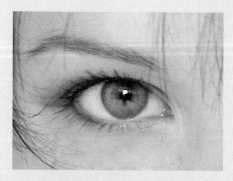

① After applying foundation to the sockets to aid eyeshadow adhesion, apply a light base over the socket up to the brow, then curl the lashes.

② Brush or sponge on a darker colour over the socket line alone and blend it. Apply eyeliner pencil to the outer tops of the lids and lower lids and blend with a sponge.

③ Apply a heavy coat of mascara to the top lashes and a lighter coat to the bottom lashes. Finish with a light blusher and neutral lips to create a daytime look.

## CREATE EVENING EYES

Life begins after work! Any make-up look goes in the evening but just remember to go a little heavier than the day for the impact you want when the light fades and the sun goes down!

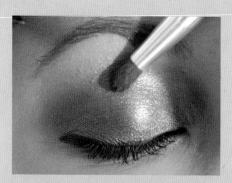

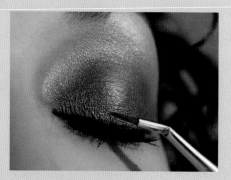

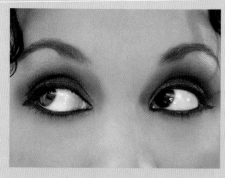

① Use a very light white or pale colour base on the lid. Highlight the upper outer brow all the way to the arch. Apply a darker colour to the socket and blend to cover the lid down to the lashes.

② Apply liquid liner to the upper lids and stretch the line just past the outer edge of the lids.

③ Apply pencil liner to the bottom lids and inside. Blend for a soft finish. Apply mascara to the top and bottom lashes, applying a little more to the top lashes to open up the eyes or apply false lashes for greater effect. A dramatic lip colour with lots of gloss or sparkle will set this look off perfectly.

# how to...

## CREATE PARTY EYES

Gloss, shimmer and shine are the way to go partying so try these shadows in any colour after applying the usual foundation base.

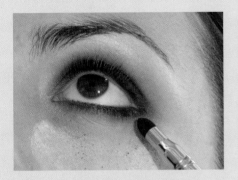

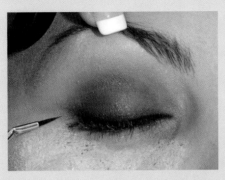

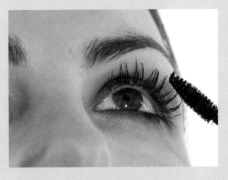

① Smudge in colour liner or a smoky grey or plum along the top and bottom lashes to deepen the effect of the overall look.

② For a really dramatic effect, apply a thick line of dark liquid liner to the tops of the lids.

③ Apply lashings of mascara in a similar way to the evening eyes but vamp up with false lashes for the wow factor!

## Contact me!

With the modern innovation in contact lenses you can really make your eyes stand out dramatically whether you are a glasses wearer or not! Gone are the days of dripping food dye into lenses and popping them in, nowadays there is a funky array of colours and designs to choose from. Some can look on the freaky side but they are fun and if attention is what you are looking for, then go for it!

Remember to match the lenses to your look and always thoroughly clean your lenses if you wish to use them again. Never use other people's lenses as this will be a recipe for bacteria-ridden red eyes.

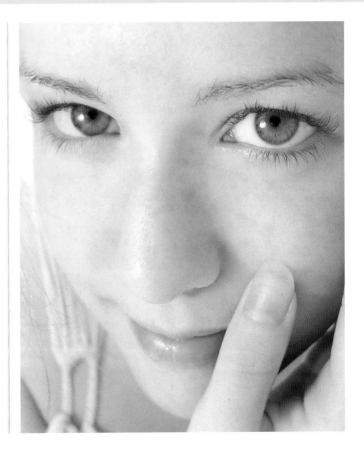

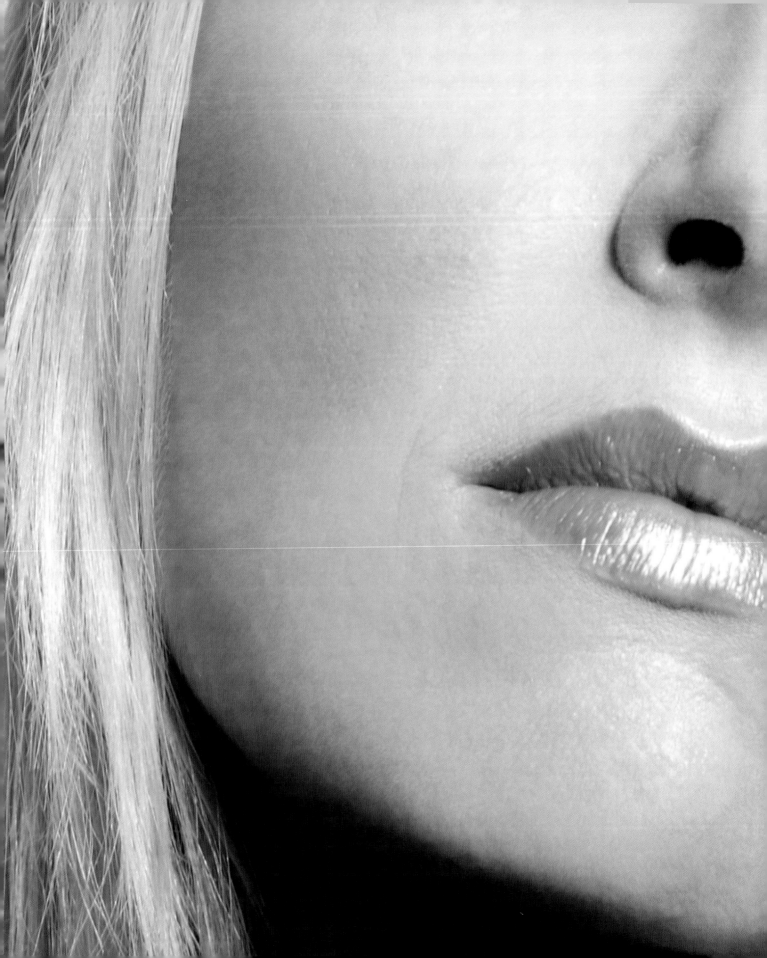

# 07 cheeks

# cheeks

Blushers are used to brighten the appearance of the face and to impart a healthy, glowing look. Having naturally red cheeks is not a reason for not wearing blusher; but having the freedom of covering the natural redness with foundation and then adding colour gives us control over where the colour shows. It is possibly the best anti-ageing cosmetic as it brightens dull skin, hiding dryness and imperfections.

When people look at you they have an instant perception; we use blusher to make sure the first impression is of health and vitality as opposed to dullness and lifelessness. Choosing a blusher colour and shade that works for you can be a minefield. With so many available on the market, which one will bring out the glow in you?

## Types of blusher

Modern blushers come in many textures and colours to create looks to suit different occasions. The lighter the product the sheerer the appearance so for a natural look go for liquids, gels and creams; for a more defined look, powder is the best option.

### POWDER BLUSHER

By far the most popular blush choice, powder is applied in sweeps from the centre of the cheek to the ear and blended using a circular movement to soften any harsh edges. Any skin type is suited to powder blush but dry or oily skins will look even better with a cream or liquid formulation.

### CREAM BLUSHER

Cream blusher is good for all skin types, especially those that require little or no foundation as this can be difficult to blend on heavily powdered skin. Mature and dry skins will benefit from the use of cream as its consistency is ideal for not sinking into lines and wrinkles! Apply to the apple of the cheek and with fingers blend out to the side of the face. Creams often give a healthy shiny finish which is unique to this product and looks incredibly natural and sheer.

### GEL AND LIQUID BLUSHERS

Excellent for a natural make-up look and those wearing little or no foundation. Both gels and liquids stain the cheeks for a sheer but colourful finish. Be sure to wash your fingertips after blending as they will stain your fingers too! Try not to drip these products – the last thing you want is blusher on your evening dress or chin! Oily, youthful skin combinations are really suited to these formulations as they are light and easy to manipulate and blend.

## Colour wash

When choosing a colour for your skin tone don't be overwhelmed by the dense pigmentation facing you in the package. Blusher is used a little at a time but is packaged to maximise quantity so often the colour you see in the packaging is a very strong version of the effect you will see on your face. Start by assessing your skin colour to see which shades will look scrumptious on you.

★ Peaches and pastels suit light and olive tones adding a sprig of youth and freshness to the face.

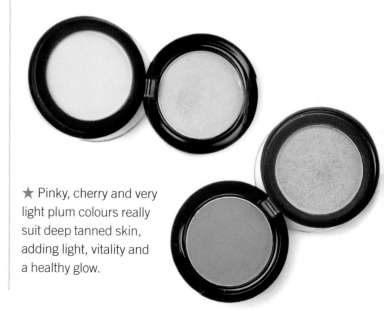

★ Pinky, cherry and very light plum colours really suit deep tanned skin, adding light, vitality and a healthy glow.

★ Blushers with a gold shimmer or a dark plum finish are luscious on medium to dark coloured skins as they freshen the face without the fear of an ashen appearance which some blusher ingredients can leave.

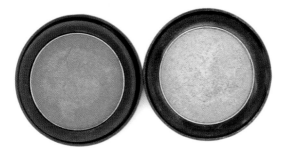

★ Bronzes and orange tones are great for darker skins of colour as they give a wonderful sun-kissed glow and illuminate the skin.

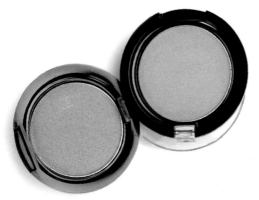

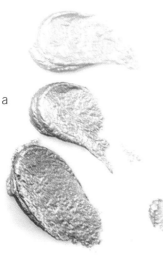

If you would like your cheekbones to be more prominent the easiest and best trick is to highlight the top of the cheekbones with a powder or cream a shade lighter than the blush and then blend down into the blusher. This looks great on all skin tones and really makes your cheeks stand out.

## The palette

Use a sponge or blusher brush which when splayed out on the cheek doesn't cover too big an area. Soft bristles are useful and a round finish is very easy to work with.

Translucent powder is great to have on standby as it diminishes intense colour should you apply too much blusher and also helps eliminate noticeable lines for seamless blending.

### COSMETICS UNMASKED

Blusher preparations are usually made from a mix of minerals such as talc, kaolin and calcium which help achieve a matt finish and offer adhesion to the skin. Blushers containing zinc and titanium are perfect for covering lined skin and expression lines, and due to their high mineral base most powders have fewer preservatives as dangerous microbial particals cannot live in a high mineral environment and are destroyed on contact with the product.

# Sun kissed

Most blushers are pigmented with peach, pink or brown tones and choosing a colour is a question of trying several out and deciding what you like best. Paler skins tend to suit a peachy, pinky blush and darker skins a plum, bronzed tone but there are no hard and fast rules; try before you buy and buy what you like!

Bronzers are now a huge best seller for most cosmetic firms and these to come in gels, powders, creams and liquids. Follow the same application rules as blusher but be warned that bronzers will be more obvious so start with a very small amount and gradually build up the intensity.

Bronzing balls are just powder in balls so if you like this idea try them out but be careful to tap off the excess or you may find a ball gets trapped in the brush and as you apply it will draw a big brown line on your cheek! These bronzers usually carry shimmer particles to give a warm look to the skin so wearing them in the winter can look unnatural. A darker shade of tinted moisturiser blended with your fingers can act as a great bronzer

Iridescent bronzers are the world's eighth wonder! They can lift a face and give a very glamorous healthy glow. Apply a small quantity to the apple of the cheeks to prevent too much shimmer in one area giving the all over sweaty look! Avoid applying to the forehead, chin or nose as often these areas are naturally shiny and do not need extra help. If you are looking for a touch of Hollywood in your evening look, apply a little bronzer to the collar bone or the top of the chest as this will give an impression of healthy sunkissed skin.

## BRONZE DRENCHED

 **Light to olive skins** look best enveloped in honey/tawny shades with slight shimmer.

 **Deeply tanned skins and lighter skins** of colour suit true bronze shades adding glow and warmth.

 **Darker skins** of colour look their best in shades of true bronze and gold shimmer.

 **Very dark skins** suit metallic, shiny coppers, deep bronzes and plums with blush to add colour under the bronzer.

# how to...

## APPLY BLUSHER

Blusher should look like a healthy glow and the more blending you do the better it looks. Take time to get it right. Ensure you use a blusher brush as other makeshift tools such as cotton wool balls or powder puffs simply do not work as the pigment is too dense when applied and you will appear to have run a marathon!

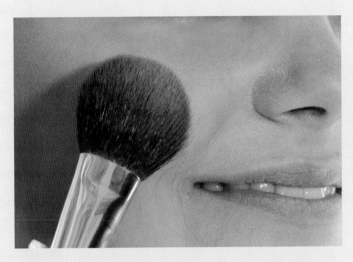

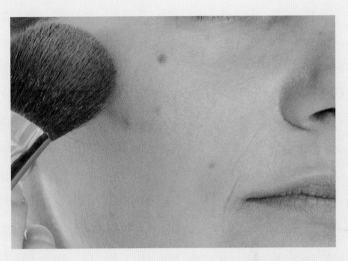

① **Smile! And the area that stands out is the 'apple' of your cheek. Apply a little blusher here to begin with and then match up the other cheek for symmetry. If using powder remember to tap off the excess from the brush to avoid too much initial colour.**

② **Blend excess product out towards your ear from the middle of the eye. If using a brush remember to dust off the excess before blending otherwise the infamous 'Aunt Sally' look could be unwittingly achieved.**

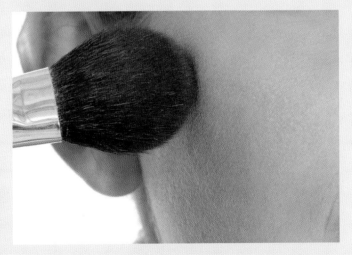

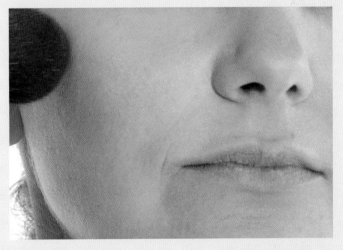

③ **With a clean brush blend in the blusher with circular movements until the edges of the colour are unidentifiable. Finish by brushing downwards to encourage facial hairs to lie smoothly on the surface of the skin.**

④ **If using a powder blush apply a little translucent powder to the finished result to reduce colour or to further blend the finished result. The illuminating look achieved gives the image of inner warmth to the cheeks.**

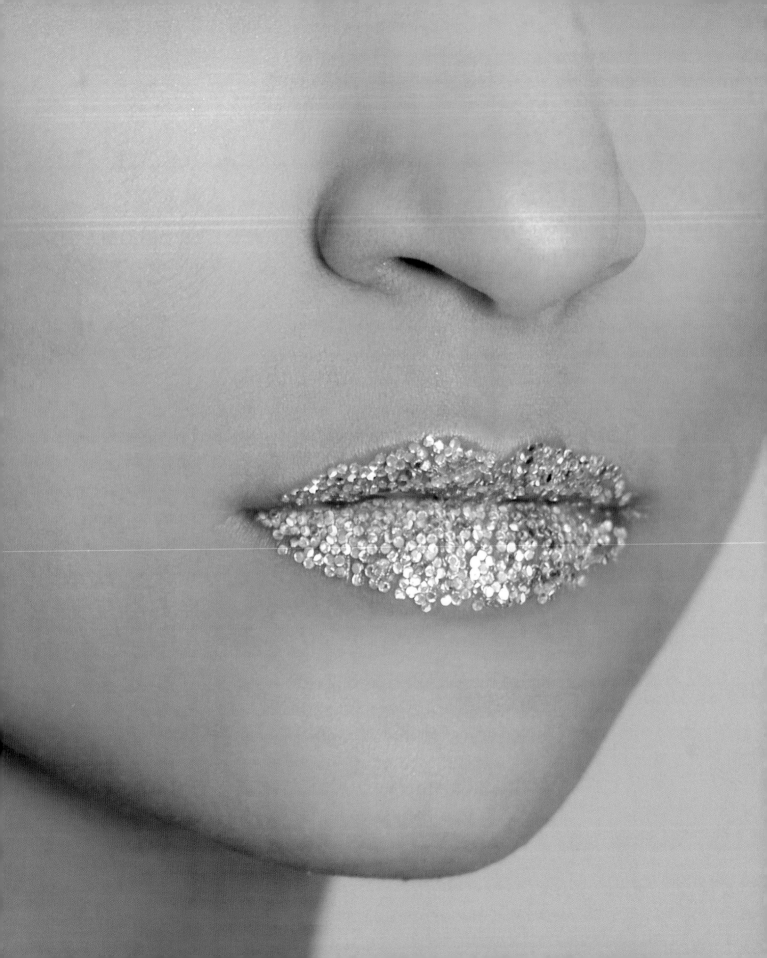

# 08 lips

# lips

Lips need to be soft and luscious in order for lipstick to really do its magic. The use of balms and gloss will help keep the lips treated and ready for the application of the most used cosmetic in the world... lipstick!

## Smoochable!

The lips are the sexiest feature of the face and in every moment in time the icons of the era have had one thing in common... a famous pout! Often people will willingly try other types of eyeshadow or blusher but not change their lipstick colour! With the wealth of colours and finishes now available, it's a shame not to try them all!

Whether you are wearing a sheer natural gloss or a bright red Monroe-style pouting lipstick all shades can suit all skin tones if applied well. Lipstick is so much fun to experiment with because it is so easy to take off!

---

### THE COLOUR FAMILY

Any lipstick you buy will fall into one of these colour categories, often though a blend of various colours is the best.

| | |
|---|---|
| ▲ Red | ▲ Orange |
| ▲ Pink | ▲ Brown |
| ▲ Purple | ▲ Beige |

---

## The perfect pout

To create the perfect look for you choose the right texture of base for your lip preparation. There are so many available you will need to assess you own lip needs and match them with a product.

Long-lasting lipsticks can be very drying even though they can last hours. Some lip stains can stay on far too long and can outlive their owners' requirements!

Matt or cream lipsticks can appear dull in comparison to their high gloss sisters but because of this dryer look they often last longer. They are unlikely to cause lipstick bleeding and are comfortable to wear because they are not slippery and great for daytime work lipstick.

Frosted or shiny lipsticks contain an ingredient called 'mica' which gives these products their shiny appearance. Usually a gloss is not needed on top and the lasting power of these products is limited to a meal or a kiss! But for the time they are on they look luscious and seductive.

Lip gloss is the ultimate finishing product for any lipstick – a high shine, short wear product which looks fantastic in any colour either on its own or over a colour base.

Lip tints are usually liquid and have a 'stained' appearance. They are super cool for a light colourful finish with no shine or heaviness.

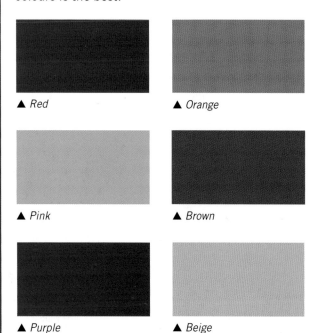

▲ Lip stain

▲ Matt lipstick

▲ Cream lipstick

▲ Frosted/shiny lipstick

## Colour me lippy

Rules are made to be broken so this simple guide can be followed or experimented with!

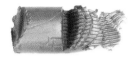

**Fair skins** looks great with a brown, champagne or pinky/peach shade of lipstick.

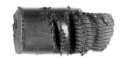

**Olive skins** suit a yellowy, brown tinge or even beige and mauves.

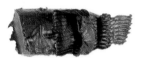

**Medium dark skin** colours tend to suit oranges, reds and burgundies.

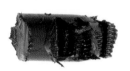

**Deeper chocolate skin** tones look great in all dark colours of red, brown and plum but can also really carry off light gloss colours.

Lips do not contain any sebaceous glands which produce the natural oils found in the skin and so can often suffer from dryness, dehydration and cracking. Protection is the key to preventing these uncomfortable and unattractive problematic pouts.

If you have chapped lips regularly apply a lip balm that contains sunblock. The sun can dry lips so be sure to offer them maximum protection from lost moisture. Also apply just over the edge of the lips to stop any further cracking of surrounding external skin.

Cold sores are created by a virus and are infectious so be sure to apply lipstick that you alone will use with a cotton bud to prevent cross infection with your fingers. If possible avoid using lipstick altogether until the area is healed, but if you must, use one that excludes pink or red tones as they will exaggerate red inflamed skin. Treating cold sores with medicated ointment from the chemist will kill the virus within days so get medicated.

## The palette

A lip brush is vital for achieving a smooth and even application to all lip preparations. Use a fine soft brush and keep it with you to touch up your lips throughout the day. If you are into changing your lip colours have a separate brush for pale colours and another for dark ones so you never have a blend of the two. Translucent powder will hold the colour in place and foundation as a base provides the perfect canvas. Lip pencils are an essential and a gloss creates the finishing touch!

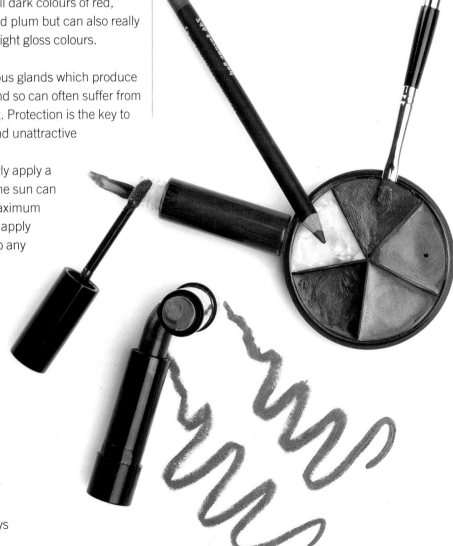

## APPLY LIP COLOUR

Basic lip colour application is easy, it just takes practice getting the lip liner right! To create the perfect base apply foundation or lip primer over the lips and a little balm if lips are dry. Starting with soft moisturised lips will only help to create an immaculate end result.

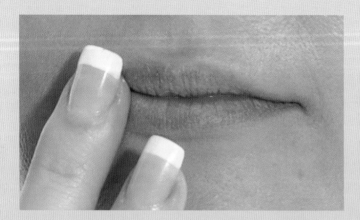

① Before applying lip liner make sure the lips are clean and well exfoliated to remove dead skin cells which cause dryness and look flaky. Remember to apply foundation on the lips to matt the surface.

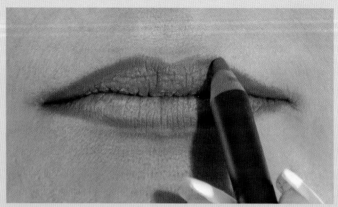

② Using a colour that mirrors that of your chosen lipstick, start in the upper central zone of the lips. This cupid's bow is the area that will be noticed by onlookers so make sure you get this right! Use a sharpened but blunted pencil and work from the centre of the mouth to the edges. Tensing your lips slightly can help even out the surface of the lips making application easier.

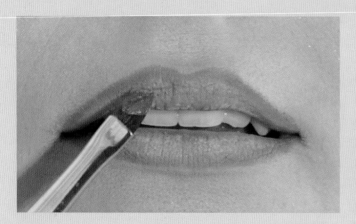

③ With a loaded lip brush follow the outside line of the lip liner and fill in the lip space. Be sure not to stretch the lips into a strange shape; a natural relaxed application will allow for a much neater result. Blot your lips when finished and apply a layer of powder over a tissue to secure the first layer.

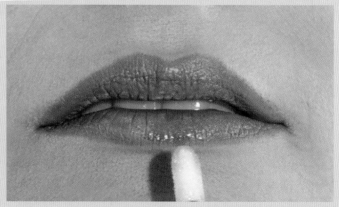

④ Reapply as above to give double protection and triple the lasting effect of your lipstick. A really good finish to the look is to reapply the lip liner to redefine the lips before applying gloss. Use the sponge wand available in the gloss product and place a dab of gloss in the centre of your lips blending out to the edges with a brush.

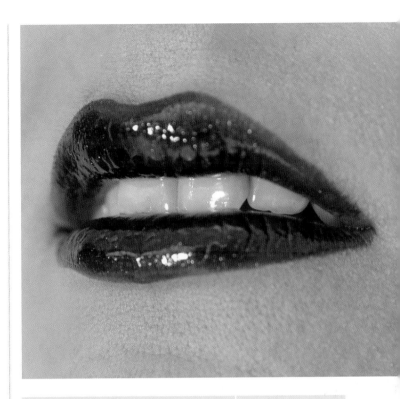

# Lip sculpture

Often one of the main complaints people have is that they are unhappy with their lip shape. Too big, too small, too thin, too fat… Although your lips will always remain that shape unless you change them with collagen injections or similar treatments there are ways to make them appear different.

### TOO BIG, TOO FULL

To minimise the look of thick lips, line just inside the natural lip line. Use a deeper shade to detract the eye away from the mouth and highlight the eyes instead. Lip gloss will make lips look bigger so if you must have shine use sheer lipstick. A clearly defined line will shrink the look of larger lips without changing their shape.

### TOO THIN, TOO SMALL

Apply a lip line to the exact shape of the lips and not over the lip line (to avoid the clown look when the lip colour eventually wears off), and fill with a medium colour. Stop just short of the corners of the mouth to give depth to the lips and add gloss for an outstanding finish. Lighter concealer round the lips can highlight the area and give the lips a larger appearance.

### MATURE LIPS

Mature lips suffer from dryness and lipstick bleeding (when lipstick seeps into the lines around the mouth). Use a lip primer to prevent seepage of pigment and line with a neutral colour. Sheer lipsticks look nice but avoid gloss! If your mouth edges turn up or down don't apply any colour in the corners and finish your application just inside the corners of the lips and mouth to detract attention away from this area.

## trade secrets

### FOR LIPS

- Use a pencil that matches your lipstick for a day look, but if you want to vamp your lips up go for a darker liner and blend, blend, blend!

- Never share lipsticks as there is a huge amount of bacteria and other germs which can be carried on lipsticks for a long time.

- Use a lip brush whenever you can as this limits the amount of lipstick you apply and makes the result last longer.

- Lip gloss makes colour look more exaggerated so use it when you want lips to look bigger.

- To prevent lipstick getting on to teeth, blot the inside of your lips with a tissue after applying lipstick.

- Try not to smudge or rub your lips together after applying lip liner and lipstick as this is the perfect recipe for ruining the look.

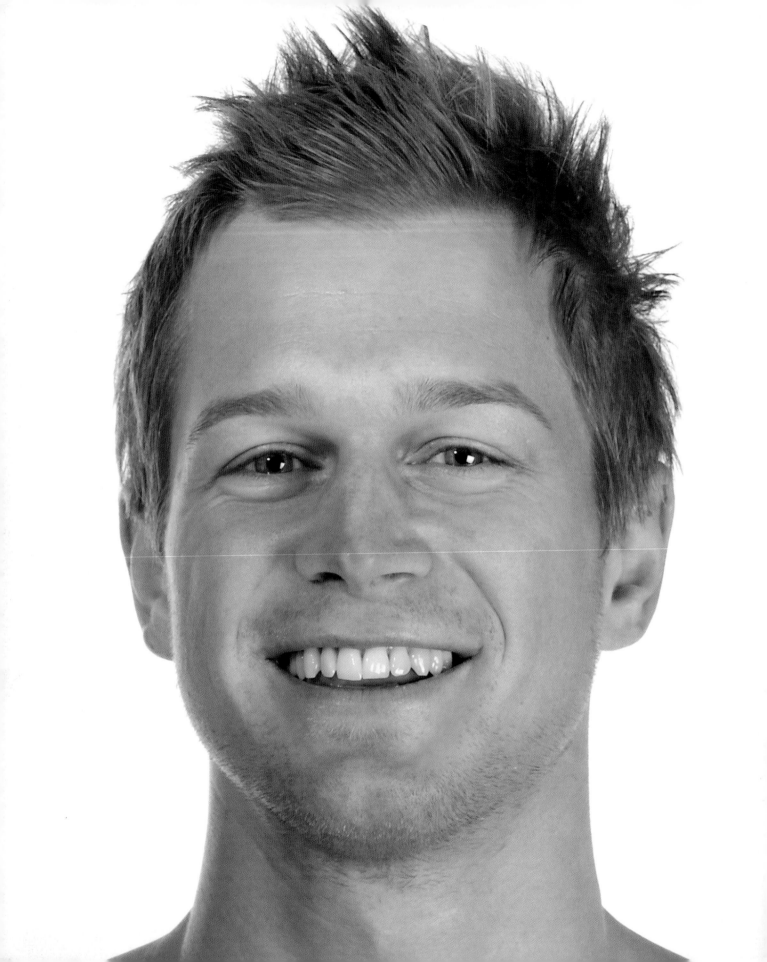

# 09 male make-up

# male make-up

A bizarre chapter you may think... But men nowadays are wearing more and more cosmetics to hide imperfections and create the look of health, vitality and good grooming! The male cosmetics market is growing year on year and men are now really looking after their skin and protecting it with SPF moisturisers as well as tinted moisturisers. Gone are the days of Mr Rough-and-Rugged! Now men also wish to achieve a brighter, healthier complexion and feel good about themselves.

Long working hours and stress contribute to skin looking dull, lifeless and unhealthy. So as well as shaving with all the latest lotions and potions, men are now looking after their skin.

## A blank canvas

It is best if the skin is in prime condition before applying any cosmetics and this requires a very clean and close shave! Although male and female skin is essentially made of the same components, it is treated very differently and this is what changes its appearance.

Male skin tends to be dryer and rougher in texture to female skin. Whether an electric or wet razor is used, the skin will still be harshly exfoliated and this is why nicks and cuts are so easy to get.

Gone are the days of using cheap throw-away razors. The more damage the skin receives over years of shaving, the older the skin will appear. These days, razors vary in shape and sharpness and there is an amazing array of different types and designs on the market which offer safety guards, multiple blades, sonic technology, pre-moisturising strips and just about anything you can think of. Using a razor that is comfortable is essential, as well as using the correct technique to shave. Guarded razors do minimise the chances of cutting yourself but do they alone provide the closest shave? Good skin cleansing and exfoliation lifts the hairs on the face and primes them for removal. So by preparing the skin well and using the best tools the shave should be clean and as close as it can be.

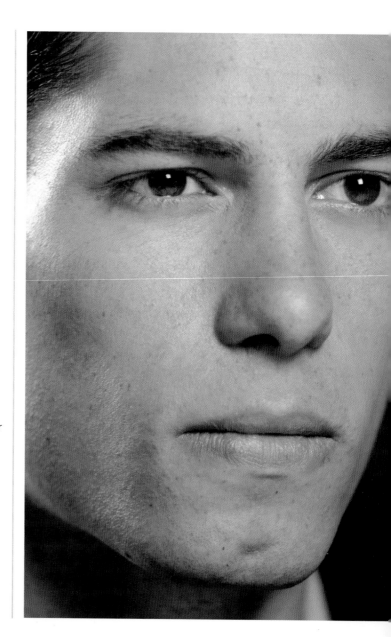

## GET THE PERFECT SHAVE

The best shave gives a clean, smooth and comfortable finish without a rash, irritation or blemishes. A good shave could also mean you reduce the need to shave daily or twice daily.

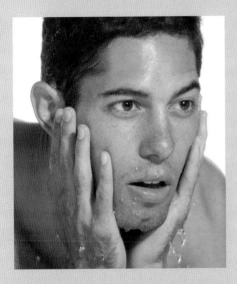

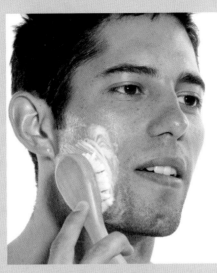

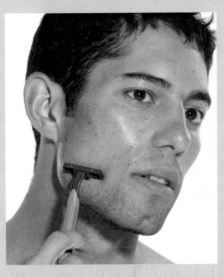

① Fill a basin with hot water and soak the razor for a few minutes to allow the metal to become flexible, making it easier to manipulate over the skin. Wet your face and apply an oil-based shaving preparation or almond oil. Avoid products containing alcohol, perfume or soap.

② Use a facial brush to lift the hairs on the face and to lather or mix the shaving product.

③ Pull the skin taut and begin shaving downwards, in the direction of the hair growth, until the whole face has been shaved.

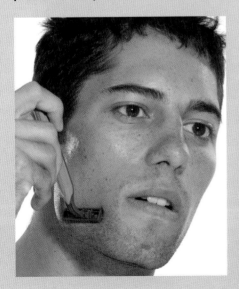

④ Now reverse the procedure and shave upwards, against the hair growth to finish, applying more shaving product if necessary. Splash cold water on the skin to remove all shaving product and wait five minutes before applying a perfume- and alcohol-free moisturiser.

### DOS AND DON'TS

✘ Do not apply aftershave on the face as this will sting and the alcohol will dry the skin and can cause an allergic reaction in the form of blemishes.

✔ Do apply moisturiser to the skin to protect it from invading bacteria and pollution that can cause ageing.

# Daily skin essentials

Every day your skin sheds millions of dead skin cells and traps pollution, dirt and damaging free radical substances on its surface. Unless these are properly cleansed away there is an increased risk of painful blemishes, dry flaky skin and blackheads.

Most men use soap and water, if anything at all, to clean their skin but there is nothing more attractive than healthy looking skin that is well cared for.

### CLEANSE

The best product to apply to the face post- or pre-shave to clean the skin is a cream wash-off cleanser. This offers the benefits of a softening cleanser, facilitating shaving whilst deep cleansing the skin at the same time. Most men prefer using just water to remove the cleanser and it is quicker, although try to avoid using a flannel as it is a hotbed for all sorts of parasites, bacteria, dead skin cells and everyday dirt. Be sure to incorporate the neck in your cleansing routine as if the area is shaved, it will need the same treatment as the face.

### FRESHEN

Using a facial spritz or toner will really brighten and freshen the skin whilst ensuring the skin's pH remains intact, protecting it from outside ravages. Use a natural alcohol- and perfume-free skin tonic where essential oils are added instead to give a nice smell without the sting! Applying it with cotton wool will leave cotton fluff on the face so either spray on and leave or slightly dampen the cotton wool first and wipe down the face so that the cotton does not get caught in the bristles of your beard.

### NOURISH

Moisturiser is essential and there are many products now available for men. If you would rather try before you buy, test your partner's or friend's moisturiser first to see what type will suit your skin. Nourishing the skin with SPF moisturisers not only protects it from the sun but shields it from everyday wear and tear and airborne scavengers that increase the signs of ageing. Aside from the external goodness, moisturising makes the skin feel soft and smooth and won't sting like aftershave. It also makes skin look bright, luminous and very kissable!

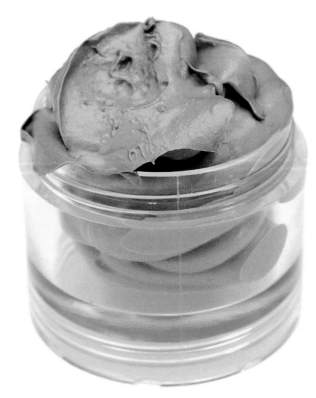

**clay mask**

# Sunday skin

Skincare routines should be quick and easy to complete. If you try using too many products you may get bored and run the risk of missing everything out instead!

Other than the daily cleansing and moisturising, it is a good idea to deep cleanse the skin with a quick facial spa once a week. The following simple routine will help to boost the skin's immunity to invading bacteria and cleanse it on a much deeper level.

### EXFOLIATION

Very gently exfoliate the skin after cleansing. It is important to use a fine-grain or small sphere exfoliant to slough off more stubborn skin cells without over sensitising the skin. Dampen the face and apply a small blob of exfoliator to the face and neck and gently circulate the product all over until a very light pinkness to the skin appears. Do not over scrub as the ensuing redness will take time to fade and is evidence of over zealous movements. Avoid the eye area as the skin is very sensitive but do incorporate the lips to eradicate roughness and flaking which can be unsightly and irritating.

## MASK

Masks can help improve the superficial appearance of the skin as well as allowing valuable relaxation time. Work out your skin type and follow the mask choices recommended in 'The Perfect Base' (see pages 32–57). Leave for ten minutes then rinse off.

Massage can also be really beneficial to skin and following the routine outlined in this book will improve the skin's circulation and toxin release systems. I do prefer to leave the facial oil on men to 'sink in' a little, as unless the skin type is oily it tends to be dehydrated and dry.

## Daily skin contouring

After shaving and cleansing it is important not only to moiturise but to use a matt lip treatment to protect lips against sun damage and possibly also an eye gel to reduce puffiness or dark circles. Modern-day male icons regularly use Botox, collagen and plastic surgery to obtain the youthful look which is so desired. By following basic skincare procedures the life of young skin will be prolonged and above all feel more comfortable to wear!

## The kit bag

The products listed below should be in every man's kit bag. Don't leave home without it!

### TINTED MOISTURISER

An ideal skin brightener without the heaviness of foundation, this light sheer consistency offers some coverage but not enough so that it is obvious. This tends to suit men by offering light coverage with the benefit of a little additional colour and a healthy glow. Wanting to cover fine lines and blemishes is perfectly natural!

### CONCEALER

Using concealer on a fully made-up face is not noticable, so use it sparingly on an otherwise unmade-up face. The trick is to use a very small amount of concealer that matches the skin colour and to blend it with a sponge to reduce the chances of unsightly lines.

### CLEAR MASCARA

Lots of women envy men and their long lashes so make the most of them and give them a wet look with clear mascara which will darken their appearance and could add even more length. Unruly brows too can be tamed to lie flat with this transparant product which simply holds the hairs in place.

### MATT LIP PROTECTOR

Lip protector is an essential smoothing and softening balm treatment, keeping the lips protected from UV light, pollutants and free radicals. It is colourless and matt and can sometimes be flavoured! Any balm is better than no balm but one designed specifically for men will ensure that it is not shiny or noticable. Cracked lips are not the best look and balms help your lips feel less dry.

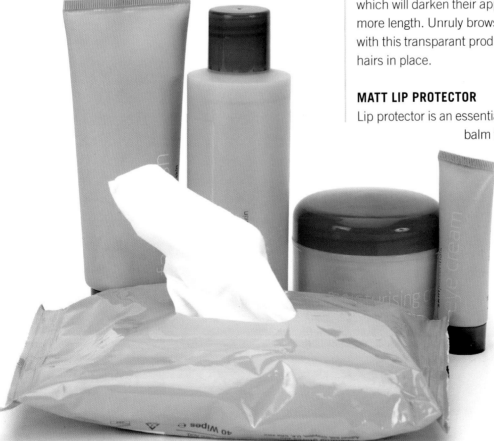

# Groom

Sometimes a helping hand is needed to achieve a groomed look. Men are now turning their attention to brows and lashes to accentuate their features. Not everyone has to turn to Botox and collagen injections but making the most of what you have can only be good.

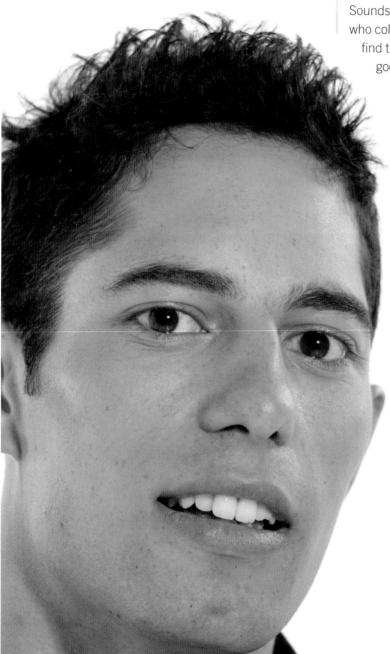

## BROW SHAPING

No, I don't mean the perfect arch! But getting rid of the 'unibrow' or odd strays can really enlarge and brighten the eyes. Concentrate on the space between the brows as this is the area where strays are noticed. Your barber probabaly trims your long brows but keeping this up yourself will only help maintain your groomed look for longer.

## LASH TINTING AND PERMING

Sounds a bit much but the result is fantastic and for those who colour their hair but don't darken the lashes you may find the two together create a more realistic look. The good thing about tinting is that it adds colour without looking unnatural, and grey or brown is often a great choice for a natural finish.

Men can follow the guidelines for facial contouring just like women to highlight and reduce areas of concern but I strongly suggest that whatever you use it should be as natural as possible.

Hair, too, can make a big difference to the face and fashion will at some point bring back the dreaded moustache! But wear whatever suits you and makes you feel confident and handsome.

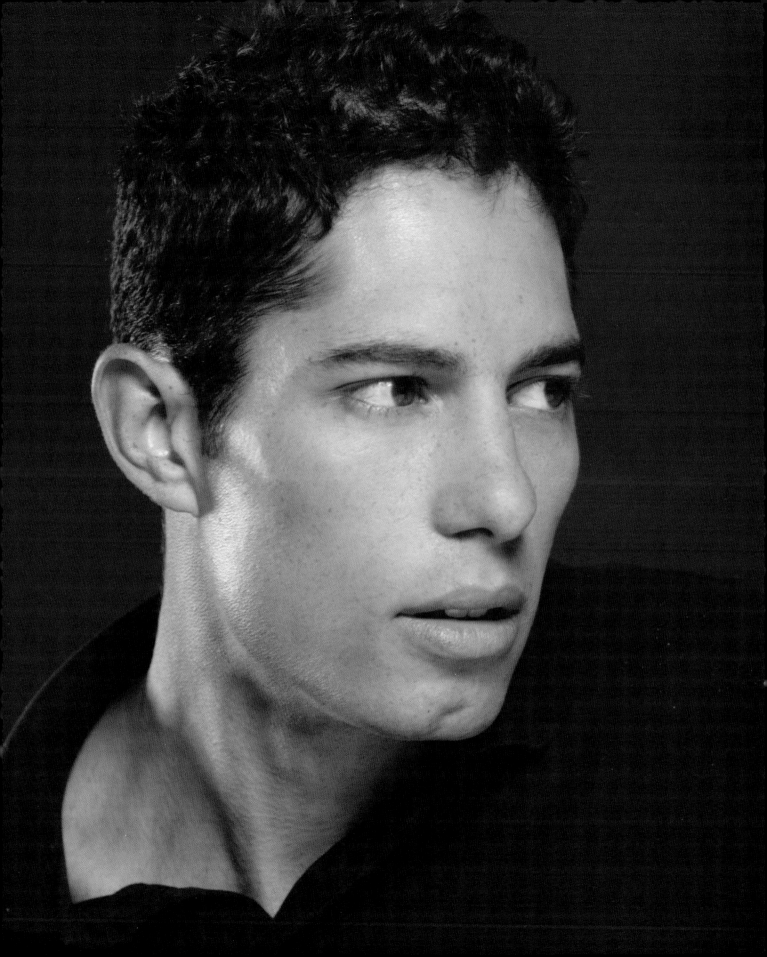

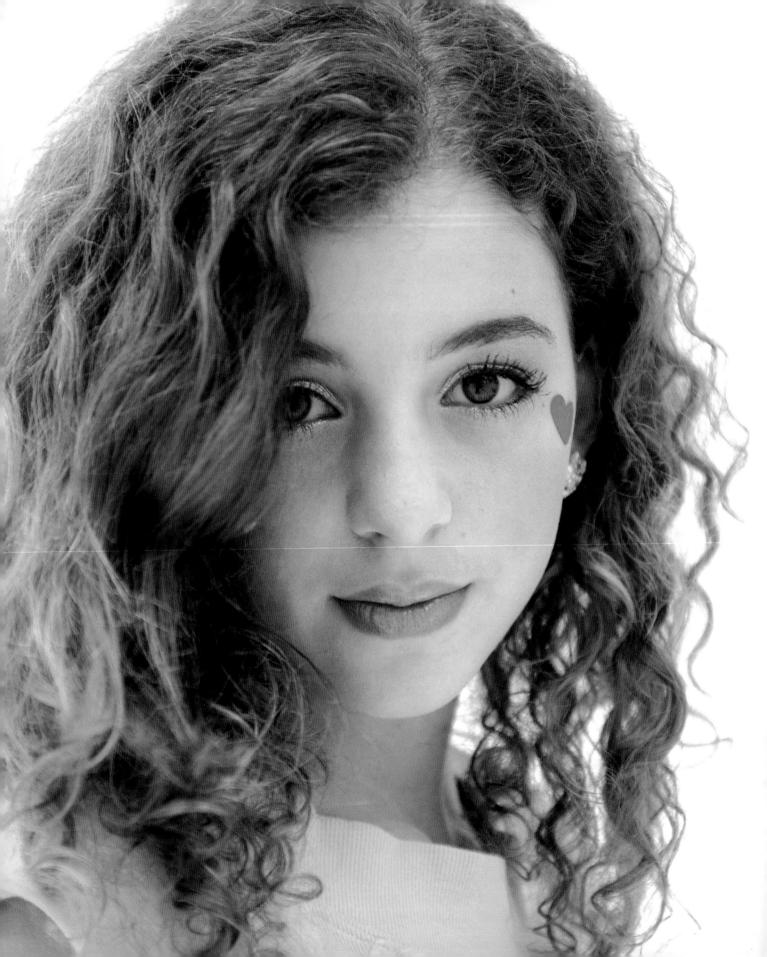

# 10 | teens

# teens

Being a teenager presents its challenges. Young skin can often be unpredictable and needs lots of care and attention. A simple daily skin cleansing regime will help you keep oily patches and blemishes under control. For those who wear make-up this chapter will offer invaluable beauty hints and tips to ensure you make the most of yourself.

## Skin solutions

During the ages of 11 to 18 the skin goes through multiple changes, from shiny and greasy to dry and flaky. This is all down to a group of male hormones called androgens which mix with the female hormones progesterone and oestrogen. Teen skin is usually greasier than older skin and is more prone to spots and blemishes, which can lead to acne. Teenage skin is very volatile and it is important to look after it through this troubled time to prevent signs of accelerated ageing and scarring from blemishes.

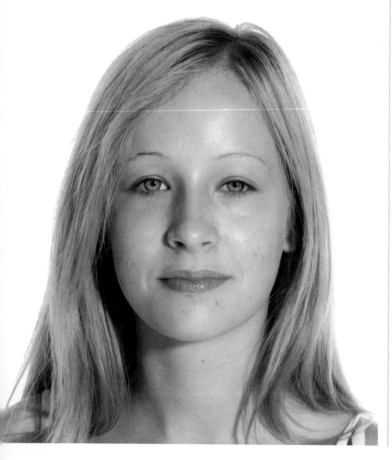

### CLEANSE

If you want radiant skin, then never pick up a bar of soap! Use products that don't strip the skin of its vital nutrients. Tea tree facial washes and cleansers are great for teen skins because they contain natural ingredients that help eliminate bacteria. Only use medicated washes for acne if they are prescribed by your doctor as these are harsh and can be harmful to the skin.

Cleanse the skin twice a day to remove the pollution, dirt, perspiration and parasites that can cause spots. Avoid using a flannel or sponge as these harbour all sorts of undesirables!

Do not saturate the skin with products containing alcohol to treat blemishes. Alcohol-based products are very strong and strip the skin of its oils which sounds great but will simply make the skin produce more oil to compensate for the loss! Cleansing wipes and teen skin products can contain these harsh ingredients so go with a natural choice like tea tree or lavender.

### TONE

For that squeaky clean feeling, use an alcohol-free toner to remove all traces of cleanser. Avoid alcohol like the plague as this dries the skin and encourages more sebum production to rebalance the skin's surface. Strong chemicals are too harsh for this young skin. Try mineral water to freshen the skin after cleansing.

### MOISTURISE

Always protect the skin from an early age by using a moisturiser with a SPF. Sun rays cause wrinkles, pigmentation irregularities, moles and even skin cancers. Moisturising the skin, even if it is oily, will create a matt feeling but provide necessary protection from the sun throughout the day. Use a water-based product and it will simply sink into the skin so you won't even know you are wearing it.

## The sizzler

Suntan lotion doesn't stop you going brown, it just prevents you from burning! So remember the golden rule: start with a high factor and gradually decrease the SPF. As you bronze, the skin becomes naturally protected so you can safely reduce the SPF number and tan further.

If you want to tan quickly, fake it! It's much safer and fake tans these days look really natural. If you are a sun worshipper and wish to apply suntan oil to your skin to speed up the tanning process, then bear in mind that you are cooking your flesh, as the combination of extreme heat, UV rays and oil is a skin killer.

## PLUCKED AND POUTING!

The main thing to remember is that from the ages of 11 to 14 you are a teen child and growing up is fast enough without speeding it up! Tidy eyebrows if you wish but be careful as eyebrow hairs don't always grow back! So stick to a shape you can wear comfortably forever just in case!

One common mistake to make is to try to make yourself look older and often it is clear to any onlookers that this is your goal. Try not to rely on make-up for this as the results are not always successful! Make-up, fashion and beauty should be fun, so enjoy experimentation without overstepping the boundaries!

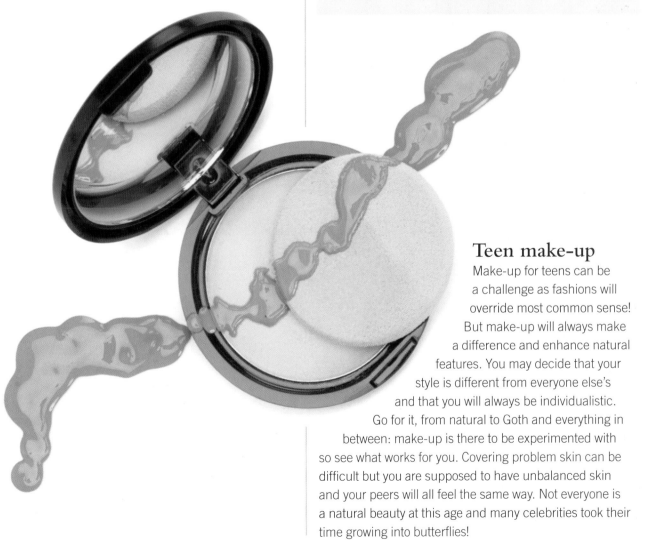

## Teen make-up

Make-up for teens can be a challenge as fashions will override most common sense! But make-up will always make a difference and enhance natural features. You may decide that your style is different from everyone else's and that you will always be individualistic. Go for it, from natural to Goth and everything in between: make-up is there to be experimented with so see what works for you. Covering problem skin can be difficult but you are supposed to have unbalanced skin and your peers will all feel the same way. Not everyone is a natural beauty at this age and many celebrities took their time growing into butterflies!

# how to...

## CREATE TEEN MAKE-UP

The most fun aspect of make-up when you are in your early teens is that you can wear anything and get away with it, especially colour, glitter and shimmer so try as many combinations as you like and have fun with trying new ideas!

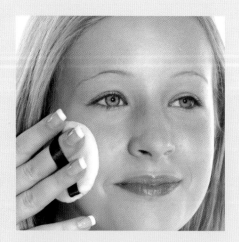

① **Start with the basics and after cleansing and moisturising prepare a good sheer foundation base and apply with fingers. Avoid the 'tide mark' by sponging in the line and blending to perfection.**

### TEENTASTIC!

If your skin is a little red or sensitive pick a base that contains lavender or other essential oils that help soothe the skin. Green concealer can cover redness but use it on larger areas as opposed to individual spots. Concealer that is slightly darker or the same as your skin tone is best used on spots and blemishes so dab a bit on with a cotton bud and blend if necessary into the foundation. Powder can look unnatural and cake-like so avoid using it opting instead for a lighter, sheerer finish.

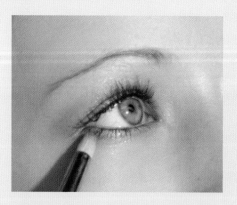

② **For the eyes try any style that suits you, but simple always has a stunning result and lasts longer. Try a light colour shadow and apply it to the lids and under the eye. Match this with a shimmer or glitter colour liner to frame the eyes for a party look and feel.**

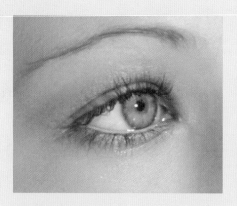

③ **Mascara and eyebrow pencils are usually not needed but use if you wish and always curl those eyelashes to open the eye and really show off the make-up!**

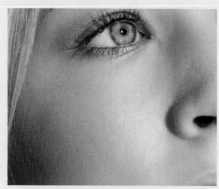

④ **Blusher and bronzer are fun additions and you should use them naturally. Cream blush looks great on young skins and the redder the natural complexion, the peachier the blush should be. Always apply to the apple of the cheeks for a fresh, healthy glow.**

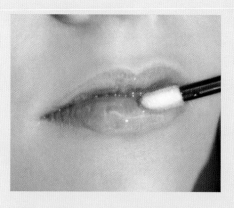

⑤ **Lipstick does not require lip liner as it will make you look like a doll! So a natural or shimmer gloss will work beautifully and really stand out!**

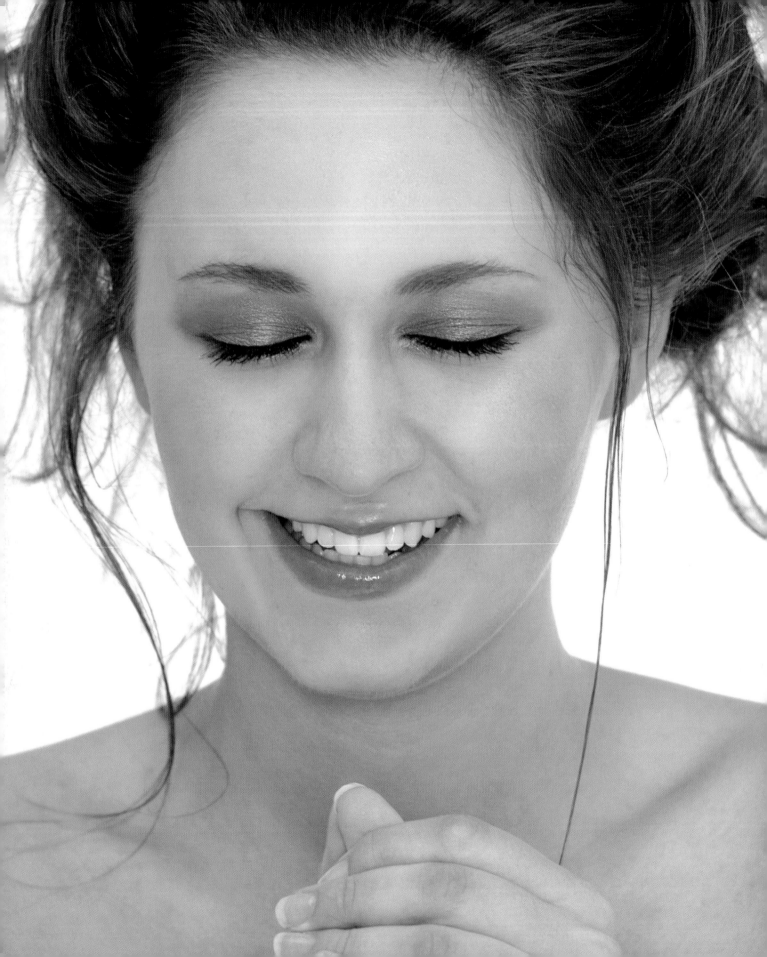

# 11 lighting and the professional choice

# lighting

Make-up can be life changing and people can sometimes be nervous about altering their appearance. When make-up artists decide on what look to choose for you they will often ask you questions about what you like, what you do for a living, what you think your best/worst features are and what the occasion is. All this information helps them decide what colours and style will work for you.

Where you apply your make-up makes a big difference to the end result and I am sure we have all come out after a department store make-over looking like a waxwork model! The lights are so strong that they change the natural

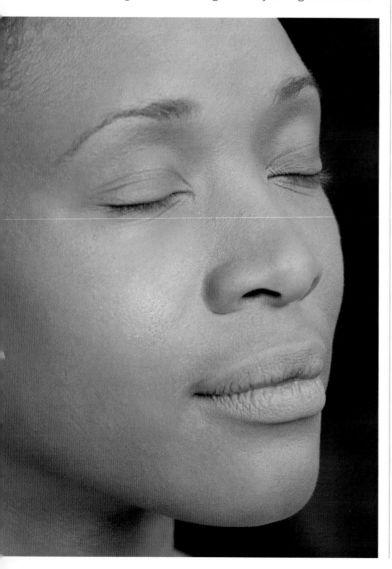

colour and tone of your face so when returning to reality the results can look rather alarming!

After a magazine or film make-up shoot I often beg the client to remove their make-up when the session is over because although the studio lights give a flawless look, it is a very different story in the cold light of day! The correct lighting is vital to achieve a professional application and here is why.

## Day make-up

Natural light is the light you are in the most so for day make-up you should apply it in front of a mirror by a window with no shadow, if possible. Often bathrooms or bedrooms are ideal as your tools are at hand, and with no artificial light disturbing the tones of the skin you will look exactly as you do in the mirror as you do outside. Carry a basic make-up kit and a pocket mirror with you to reapply your make-up throughout the day.

I often see people taking this one step further and doing their make-up in the car and on the bus or train! This is not advisable for obvious reasons! Set some time aside and do your make-up properly. This will save you time in the long run as you won't have to correct mistakes or touch up your make-up as regularly.

## Photographic make-up

In a studio artificial light is used to create a flawless image. Nearly all photographers shoot digitally now as the pictures can be easily changed and deleted. This includes 'touching up' areas which are not quite so flawless! Lighting takes time to get just right and often photographers use black or white backgrounds to absorb or reflect light where it is needed. Studio lights are very strong and make-up needs to be able to swim rather than sink so applying extra

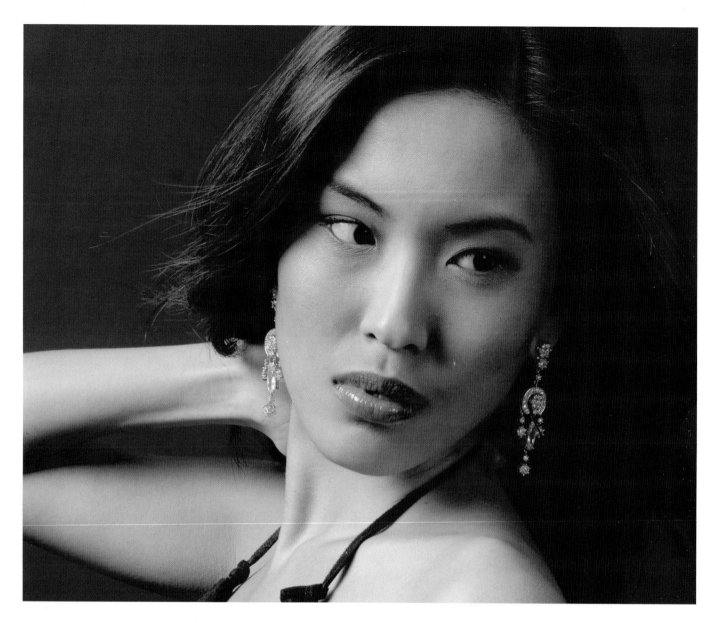

everything is essential. Often women and men feel plastered with make-up but it is really important to understand that your make-up artistry will be devoured by the light if not applied properly.

## When the sun goes down

Dark rooms and dark lights fool us into thinking imperfections cannot be seen but when the dreaded flash photography starts we are suddenly plunged into bright light and everything is captured! The trick is not to go heavier on foundation, concealer and powder just because it is night time but to go a little heavier on the eyes and lips instead.

## Wedding make-up

Wedding make-up is tricky to master and many brides have their make-up done professionally for their big day. During the day, a light and natural look is best and adding to your make-up for the evening will ensure you look just as good after hours.

My years of experience in this field have taught me that the worst mistake to make is not to book a trial run-through with your make-up artist. Don't run the risk. Both artist and bride must be satisfied with the look before the big day.

Weddings are stressful and so make-up artists need to be aware that extra patience, understanding and calm are all professional qualities that need to be brought to the fore.

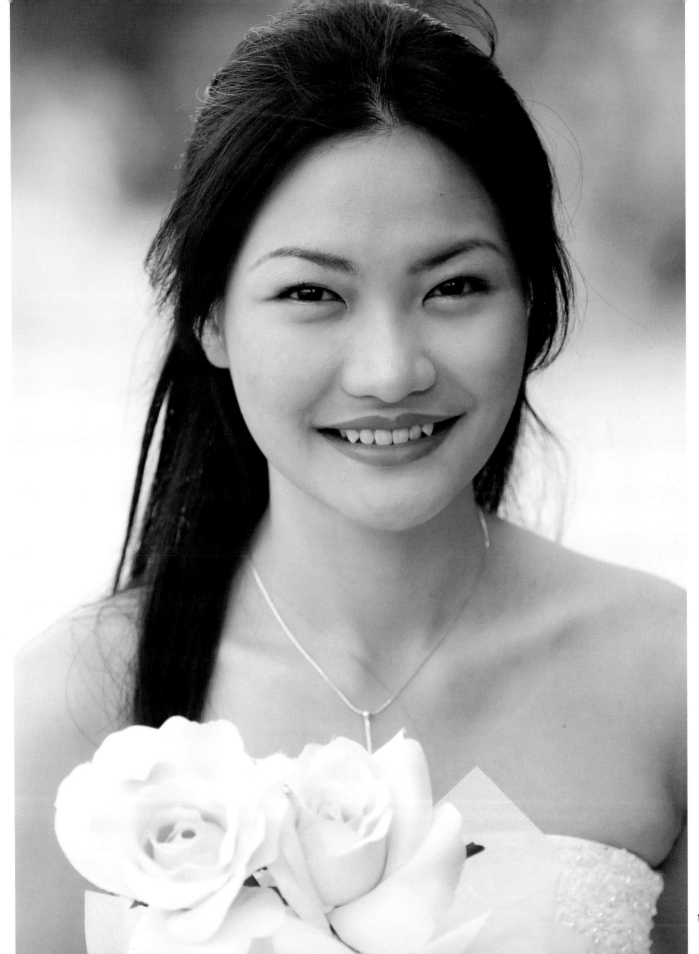

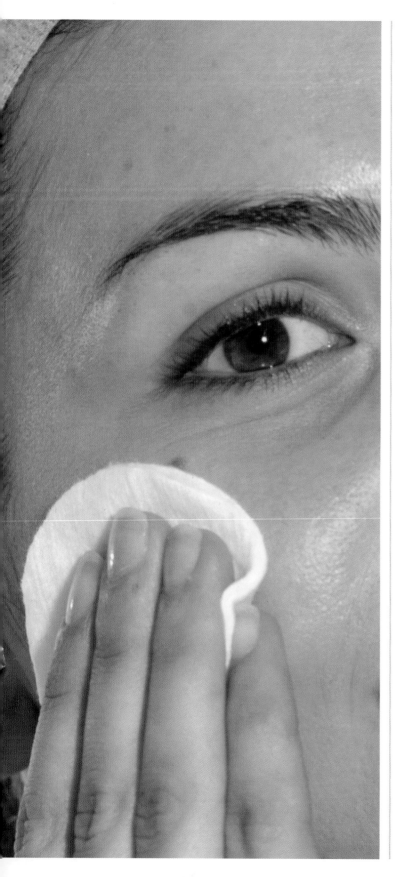

## The professional choice

I have been asked many times to give product advice by all types of men and women wanting to make better choices for their skin. It is not always easy to pick key products from such a vast selection and it can be daunting when cosmetics companies advertise a multitude of liposomes, plumpers and exotic plant, fruit and marine extracts!

## The right choice

Skin care and make-up choices should not totally be based on price as the most expensive brands are not necessarily the best. Never be fooled by beautiful packaging and expensive marketing campaigns! Cosmetics companies around the world use a plethora of slogans and celebrities to sell their goods. It's an approach that sells as we all want to look, or feel that we can look, like our favourite celebrities.

To me skin is about both nature and nurture. Nature gives you good or bad skin genetics – looking at your parents will give you a pretty good idea what you will look like when you are older. Nurture is how we look after our skin. People with weak skin genes can have beautiful skin but it does take time and energy to keep up this level of care. It's not about being vain or affected but about being healthy and caring for what nature has given you.

So many people have asked me for anti-ageing products when they already have copious amounts of lines and wrinkles! Making the effort when you are young is essential.

## Don't be lazy!

The following list dispels some of the myths surrounding products from skincare to make-up. Don't forgo your daily skin routine – it's worth the effort!

### CLEANSERS

These are always water- or oil-based. Even though water-based cleansers are good for oily skin, oil-based ones remove make-up much more effectively. Wash-off cleansers do not remove make-up thoroughly and hard water can make the skin feel tight. Some cosmetics companies only have one cleanser for all skin types which can feel like your specific skin type is not being treated, but remember, cleanser is only on the skin for a few moments to remove make-up and pollutants – it is not made to treat the skin.

As always avoid highly perfumed and preserved cleansers as these can cause skin reactions. It is worth spending a

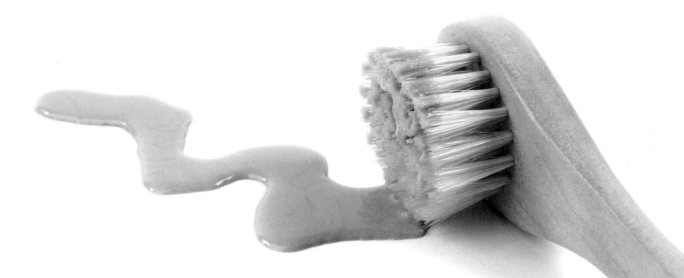

little more on a cleanser as the cheaper ones are quite basic. Facial wipes and two- or three-in-one products do not work as they seem to take a long time to do just one job (cleansing) let alone three (toning and moisturising)! Don't cut corners and make sure you use the right products!

## TONERS

Toners are quite often underrated but they are great for making you feel fresh and revived. Don't spend a lot on a toner as its main ingredient is water with a few extra ingredients such as plant or fruit extracts to perfume the product but also to treat the skin and rebalance its surface giving that squeaky clean feeling. Go for a natural floral water to remove traces of cleanser and to freshen the skin. Some toners have a high alcohol content which dries out the skin so opt for a more friendly version with a low alcohol content to really boost surface hydration.

## MOISTURISERS

Most people moisturise on some level and most understand the benefits of hydration. But are we paying too much? The answer I have always given is use what you enjoy using. Moisturisers will stay on the skin so pick one that feels comfortable and nourishing without adding too much oil to the skin. Always use a moisturiser with an SPF and don't be conned by reams of wonderful sounding ingredients as these can be present in very minimal quantities. Instead opt for one you can afford and like the consistency of as this will feel good on your skin and encourage you to use it regularly. Natural extracts such as essential oils, herb and plant extracts can be great skin boosters so your choice should mirror your skin's needs. Always ask advice from a beauty therapist if unsure what to purchase.

Moisturiser has two basic functions: to protect and to nourish. Just because a moisturiser suits your best friend it doesn't mean it will suit you so try out a few samples first. The best selling moisturiser in the world is bright yellow and sells like hot cakes! But is it any good or is it just great marketing? Celebrity endorsements can be useful but often celebrities are given free products to try and are photographed carrying them. For all we know, they might be carrying them to the skip when the paparazzi catch them on camera! Make-up artists do not tend to use expensive moisturisers on their clients as they do not stay on the skin long enough. The more ingredients a product contains, the more chance your skin has of reacting so bear this in mind.

# Skin treats

Every so often the skin needs a pick-me-up treatment to give it freshness. In the winter months the skin can appear dull and dry so a serum or liquid peel treatment can refresh and boost your skin's texture and glow.

## EXFOLIATION

Exfoliation is the best for sloughing off surface dead skin cells. There are many types on the market but I find the fine grain ones best as they buff the skin rather than scratch it. Large nut particles in cheaper products can be very harsh on the skin and still don't remove dead cells. Products containing 'spheres' can be technically great but are often too smooth to do any real good, so again try before you buy on the back of your hand. Liquid exfoliators and skin peels vary in strength so be sure to do yours when you have time for the skin to recover! Exfoliate twice a week for a smooth complexion or skin brush the face for a lighter exfoliation and to stimulate the lymphatic system (see page 48).

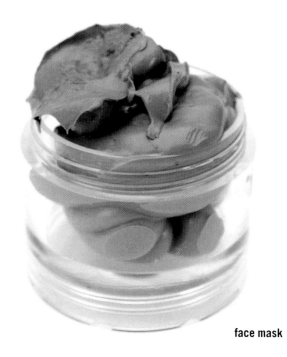

**face mask**

## MASKS

Bearing in mind that the first three layers of skin are dead, face masks are somewhat of a mystery treatment! You may find that though your skin may not look drastically different, it feels fresher, tighter and cleaner. For me masks are purely psychological nursing; they provide a much needed break for relaxation so although I may underestimate the power of the mask I will never underestimate the power of the rest! Don't overspend on masks but if you like the feeling use once a week with a mandatory cup of tea and a bath!

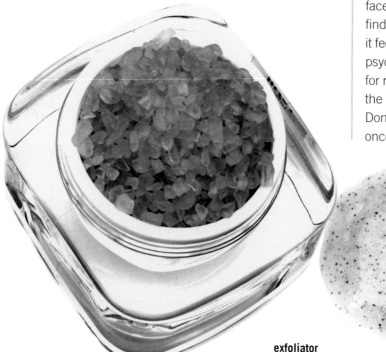

**exfoliator**

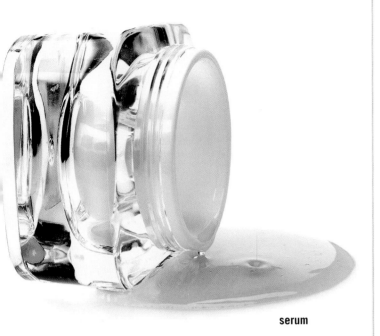

serum

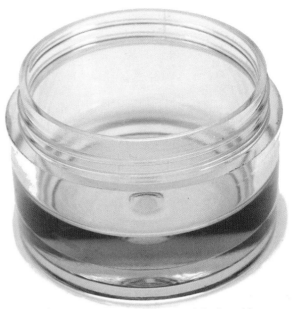

night time skin treatments

## SERUMS, AMPOULES AND LIQUID TREATMENTS

These specialist products are packed with active plant and herbal extracts to boosts the skin's appearance and texture. Serums are slightly oily and come in pump-action bottles which release the exact amount needed per application, whilst ampoules and liquids come in bottles to enable you to use as much or little as you like. Just remember these extra zesty products should be used in small doses as any more than is needed is a waste of product and money! These skin treats can be expensive so only choose ones you can afford or alternatively copy the ingredients from nature and make your own treatments from fruits, herbs and plants!

## NIGHT TIME SKIN TREATMENTS

These products can be an additional expense you don't need. Skin regenerates at night and sebum zones fill. If you over nourish the skin with heavy moisturisers in these sleeping hours you can wake up with an over oily skin that feels uncomfortable. Most skin does not need 24-hour nourishment so either ease off at night altogether as the skin produces natural oils or use a smaller amount of your normal day moisturiser.

## EYE TREATMENTS

Eye treatments work wonders. Cool eyes feel right and we could all do with a bit more vitality in the eye area to make us look awake when we are not feeling it! Eye treatments need not be expensive; pick a product you can afford to use regularly as this will benefit you a lot more. Opt for a serum or cream gel as they do not leave a tacky finish. Dab onto the eyelids and around the sockets, allowing it to soak in before applying make-up. Eye packs and masks have a temporary effect but feel like pure luxury and are an absolute must!

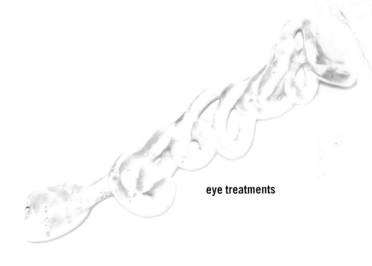

eye treatments

# Truly, madly skin deeply!

When it comes to make-up the market is flooded with enticing products, but investing a little time to choose the right ones for you will save you money and effort.

## FOUNDATION BASE

Of all the make-up products this is where your investment should lie. A good base won't be cheap but will last a few months and will ensure you look great every day. No tide marks or orange collars here! Less is more when it comes to foundation so go for a lighter coverage as this will look more natural. Whichever your texture preference don't compromise on colour tone and don't try squeezing into one of a range of four colours! If you don't find exactly what you want, have your foundation tailor-made – it may cost a little more but the result will be worth it.

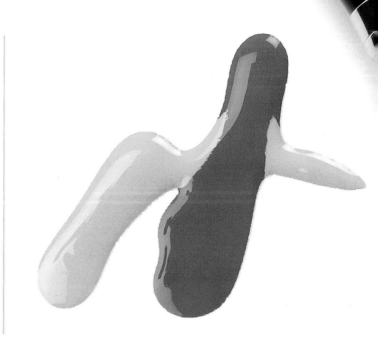

## CONCEALER

This little pot of magic should be just a hint lighter than your natural tone and applied in small quantities. It comes in many forms: cream, wax, pencil, pen, tube, block or colour wheel. You shouldn't skimp on this product; make sure you buy one that suits your needs and that is long lasting. Blemish treatments are useful because they cover spots as well as treating them. Concealer is great applied around the corners of the nose, under the eyes and in the chin crease to mask dark areas and reduce flush.

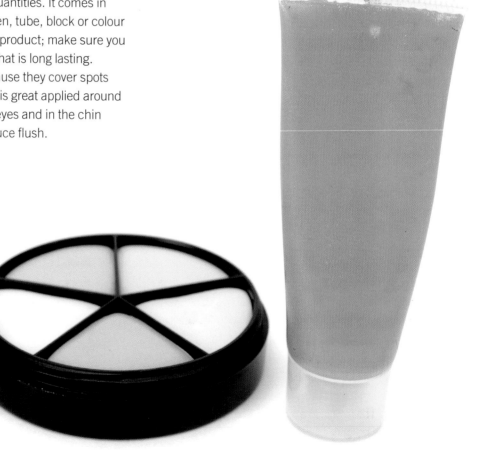

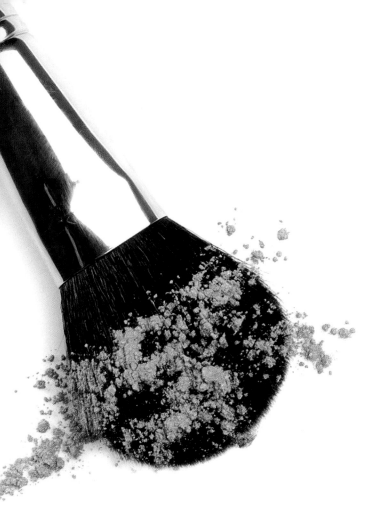

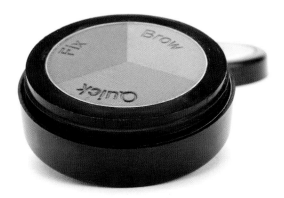

with a selection of three colours which are applied with a slanted brush. Blocks are not easy to come by, so look out for them!

## EYESHADOWS

Up until recently I would have said that anything goes but the new generation of shadows are ultra fine and highly pigmented, giving a superb finish and intense colour. Go for individual shadows – a compact with a selection of colours may not be the right choice as there will be at least one colour you won't want to wear. I still love working with powders because of their blending ability but liquid, cream and gel textures are great for achieving a more natural finish.

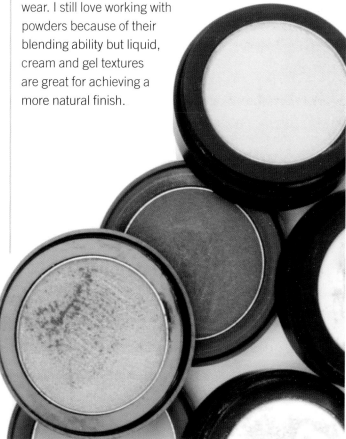

## POWDER

As long as it is translucent powder can be fairly cheap. The better powders are very fine in texture but translucent ones are invisible so they need not be so fine. More expensive translucent powders appear white but will disappear into the skin when brushed in to leave an invisible powdery finish. You need not break the bank when it comes to powder but do invest in a good quality brush to apply it. A large dome-shaped brush will disperse any powder no matter how cheap.

## EYEBROW PENCILS

These are a must to add definition and colour to eyebrows. The best ones are either soft or chubby pencils or blocks

## MASCARA

There are now many different types of mascara on the market all promising to nourish, lengthen, curl, thicken and plump your natural eyelashes, but what works best? Some leading French cosmetics companies collared the market a few years ago because their mascaras were indeed long lasting and easy to use as well as delivering upon the promise of longer, thicker lashes. However, the tables have turned and nowadays make-up artists tend to choose the cheaper brands because they are just as good and more affordable. The new trend of white building base products which are then coated in mascara do give a dramatic effect but be sure not to apply too much base as you might find it clogs up the lashes. Make sure you follow with a good coating of mascara to ensure that the white base is no longer visible.

## EYELASH CURLERS

Lash curling is essential, and a basic lash curler is affordable and creates fabulous results. Heated lash curlers do not actually curl the lashes but they set an existing curl better, so make sure you choose the right tool!

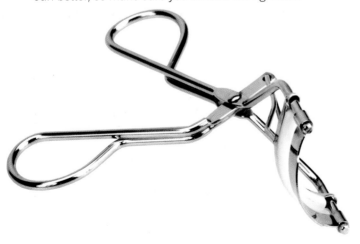

## EYELINERS

A must-have product that doesn't come cheap. Price is everything here as cheaper pencils tend to be hard and scratchy. The more expensive pencils contain creamy conditioners, are soft and slide on the lid effortlessly. Bearing in mind eye pencils last forever this is a good investment. Try pencils on the back of your hand before buying; colour should appear with the lightest touch, if you have to rub it on, don't buy it!

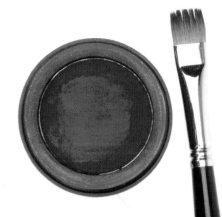

## BLUSHER

What a selection... There used to be only powder but now we are tempted by gels, creams and liquids. I have one of each for different looks, but nearly always use the same shade of colouring. Go for one or two colours that you know suit you: one for daytime wear and another slightly stronger shade for the evening.

## BRONZERS

Bronzers are great for a sun-kissed look in the summer so choose one to match your natural colouring. You should use a slight shimmer blush for a true sun-kissed look, not a shiny product, and don't go really cheap as these products are made of thicker bulkier ingredients which do not blend as well.

## LIPSTICK

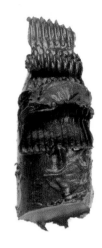

You can never have too many lipsticks! Lipsticks come in all sizes, colours and shapes, from the traditional sticks to shimmery pencils and gloss tubes. These days we want products to be compact, quick and convenient to apply. Go for a simple lipstick that contains as few ingredients as possible, especially as you will be consuming most of the daily application! Lipsticks vary enormously in price so go for what you can afford and test the texture before buying. Creamy lipsticks do not have as much staying power as the long-lasting variety which can stay on for hours on end! However, these tend to dry the lips terribly so always use lip primer or balm before and after to soften the lips and prevent flaking.

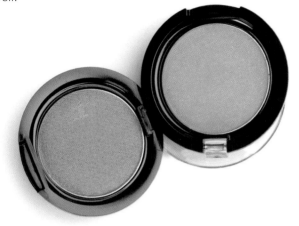

## LIP LINER

A must for the perfect pout! Like eyeliner, lip pencils should be soft and should glide on the lips. Try on the back of your hand before buying. Lip pencils are often sold with a brush on one end to help blend the lipstick to the line. Never sharpen a lip pencil to a sharp point as it will break when applying; instead sharpen and then blunt the end slightly before using. For day time wear choose a liner that matches your lipstick but why not go for a slightly darker line for evening wear to vamp up your look!

## SHIMMER AND SHINE

Glow adds a healthy sheen to the skin and suggests vitality and inner health. There are hundreds of shimmer, shine and glitter products that enhance this look and some are out of this world! Creamy combinations work well for cheeks and glitter looks fantastic on the eyes and lips. Too much shine can be overpowering so make sure you use the right products in the right areas. Adding touches of glitz and glamour to your evening or party make-up simply must be done!

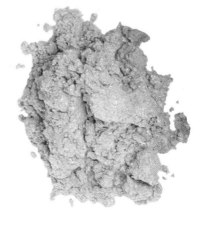

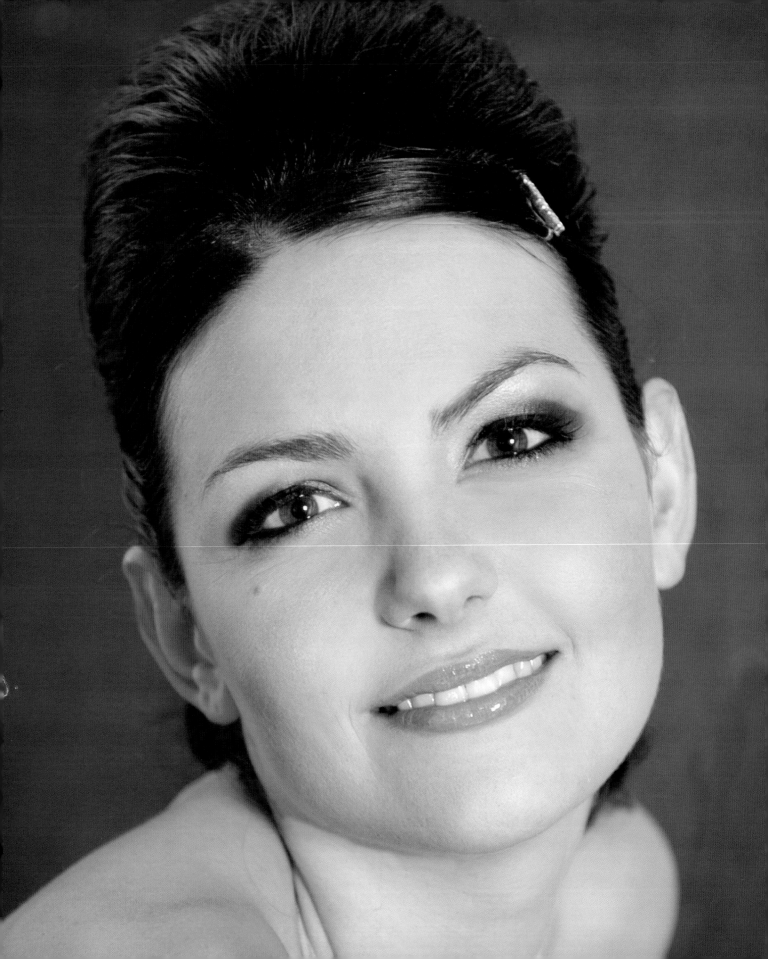

# 13 the look

# the look

Whilst fashions change with the seasons some make-up looks from history have been popular enough to keep coming back year after year. So why is that? Usually because they are simple to achieve and they make everyone look good! Underestimating the power of make-up is a mistake and stars past and present know all too well that their look could end up being the next big thing. This chapter covers the most popular looks past and present!

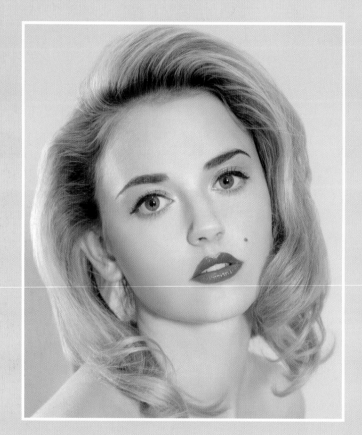

◀ **fabulous fifties**
see pages 134–137

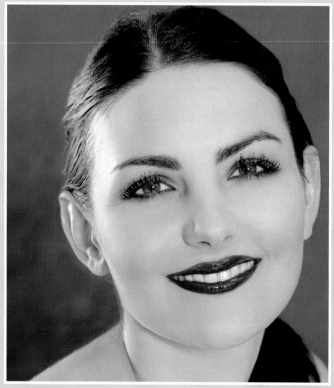

▶ **glitz and glamour**
see pages 138–143

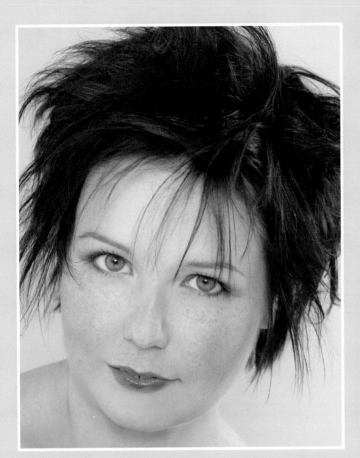

◄ **dare to be bare**
see pages 144–147

▼ **metal mania**
see pages 148–151

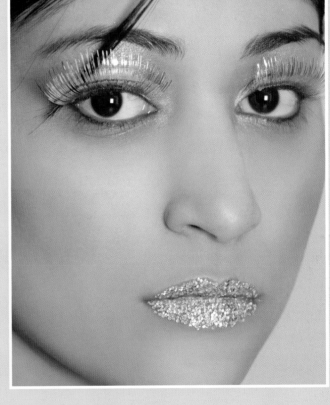

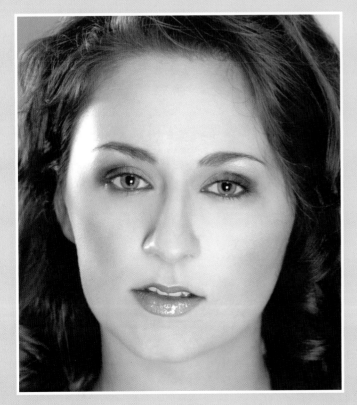

◄ **nature's finest**
see pages 152–155

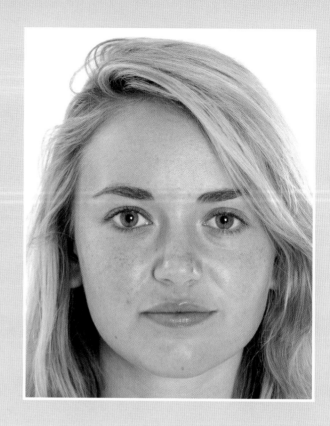

# fabulous fifties

Marilyn Monroe used a blend of white powder and Vaseline to achieve the flawless base she is renowned for. Fortunately we can achieve the same effect and increase staying power by using a combination of foundation and concealer. Undemanding make-up such as this takes little effort to apply but the trick to replicating it is in the application!

See pages 136–137 for how to create this look

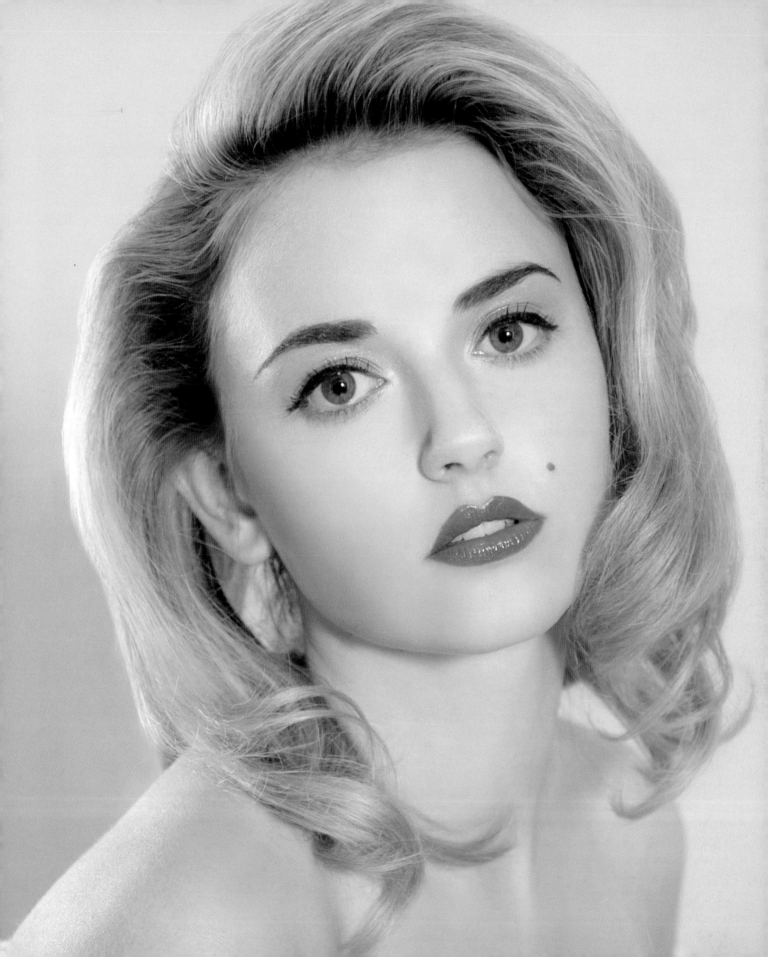

# how to...

## CREATE THE FABULOUS FIFTIES LOOK

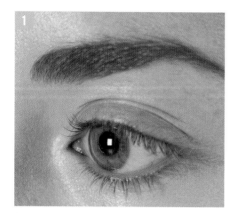

① Start by applying a medium to light sheer foundation with a sponge all over the face, including eyelids and lips. Blend the base into the neck and forehead to prevent obvious lines.

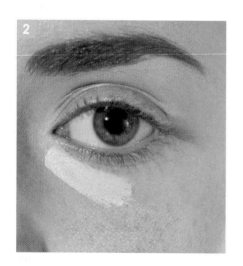

② Conceal under the eyes in a light to natural tone and reduce any redness around the nose or cheeks in the same way. Darken the brows with a brow pencil and define the natural arch of the brow as much as possible.

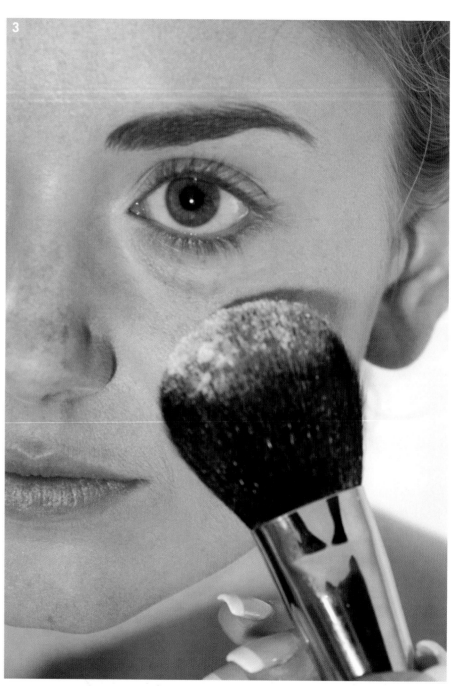

③ Dust a generous layer of translucent powder over the face to set the base and to provide an overall matt effect. The sheer foundation will complement most skin tones if this make-up changes with heat or perspiration.

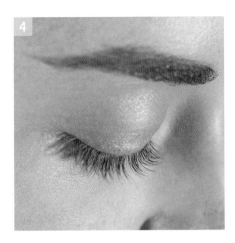

④ Apply a light creamy powder shadow to the lids up to the brows with a sponge or brush.

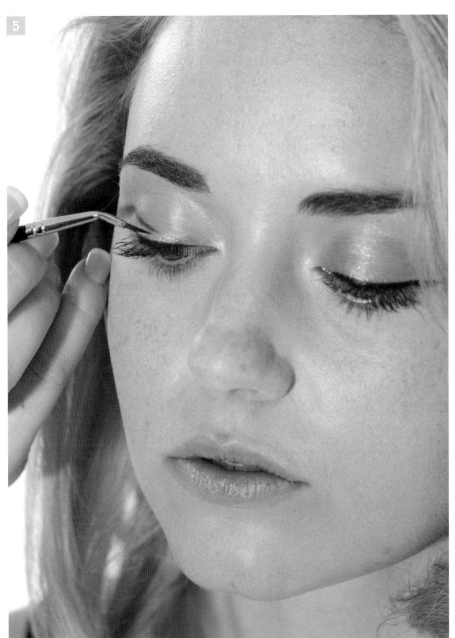

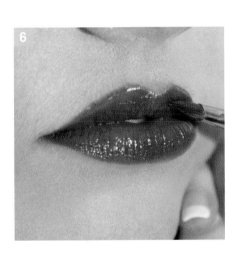

⑥ Lightly apply a peach cream blush to the upper outer cheek area, avoiding the 'apple' of the cheek to create a barely there appearance. Finally apply a deep red lip liner and matching lipstick to fill the lips and try to make them as naturally big as possible.

⑤ Apply a generous line of black liquid eyeliner to the upper lid and slightly exaggerate the line at the outer edge. For a truly stunning effect apply strip or individual false lashes before applying a generous coat of black mascara to the upper lids. A finer or clear mascara is used on the lower lashes as these are not defined.

### AND LASTLY...

Beauty spots were very popular in the 1950s so for authenticity you may wish to apply one with a black or brown eye pencil!

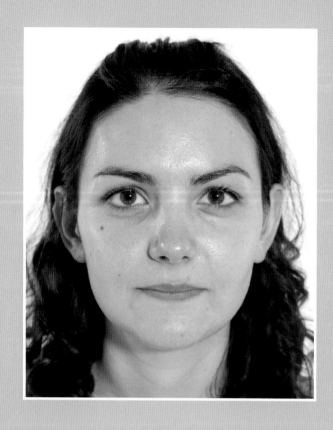

# glitz and glamour

Many make-up styles we see today are based on fashions from the 1960s and 70s. Smokey eyes and vibrant colours represented these eras perfectly and with modern twists we can create the most dramatic, sexy and sultry make-up of all time!

See pages 140–143 for how to create this look

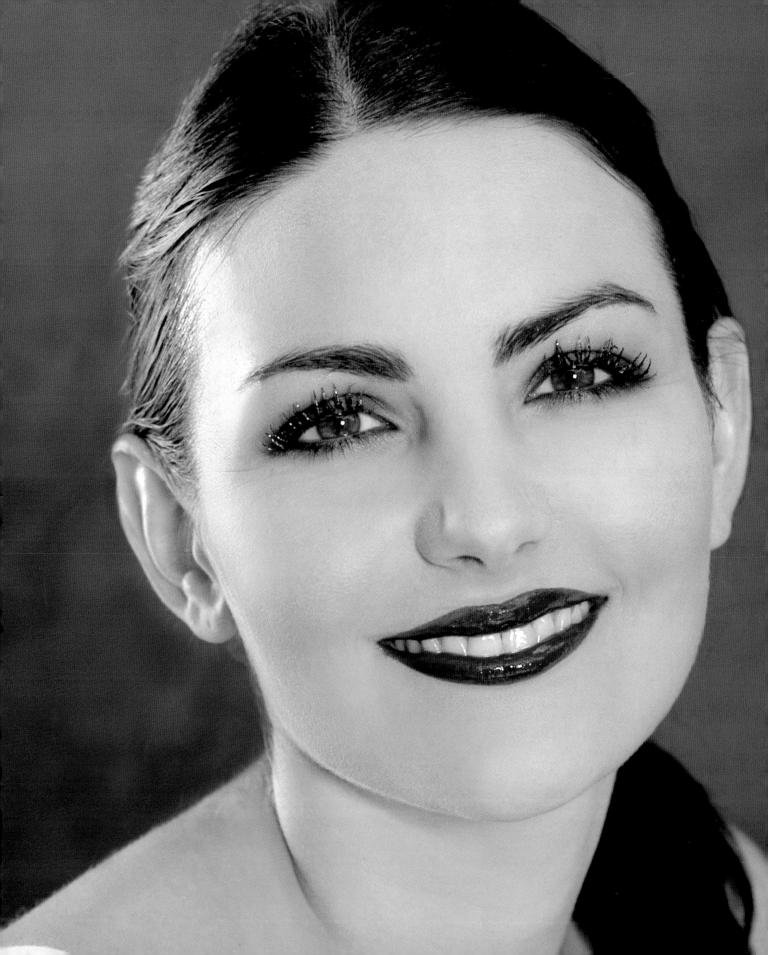

# how to...

## CREATE A GLITZ AND GLAMOUR LOOK

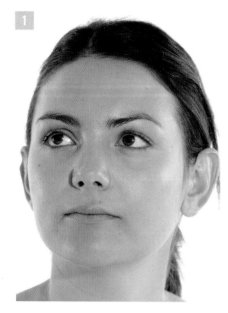

① Apply a sheer base all over the face to reflect light and give a luminous appearance to the complexion. Conceal any imperfections around the eyes and nose to complete the canvas.

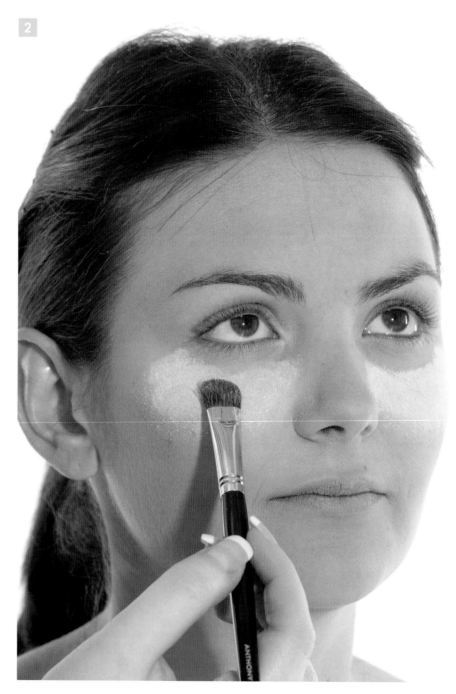

② Brush on a generous amount of translucent powder and apply an extra layer under the eye area to protect against loose particles of shadow. Any crumbs of shadow that fall on the face can then easily be brushed away without spoiling the rest of the make-up.

③ Apply a cream or white powder shadow to the whole lid up to the brow with an extra highlight in white under the arch of the brow.

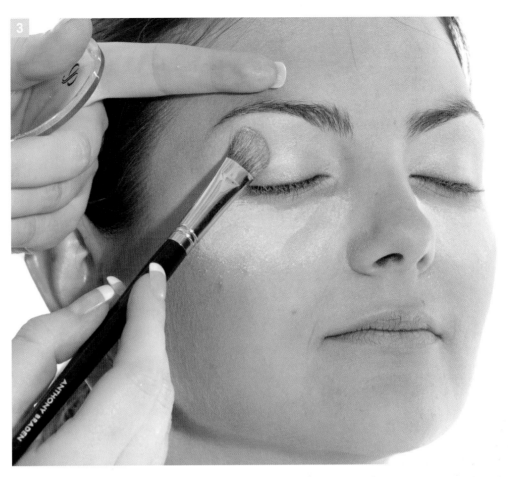

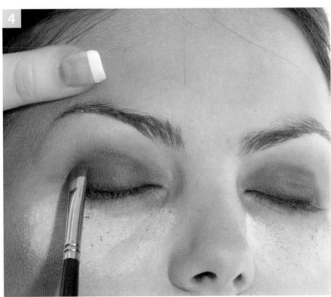

④ Carefully and slowly apply a dark grey, plum or black shadow to the lid and socket and blend to smooth the appearance of the edge line. Shadow pencils are often best here to really control the colour.

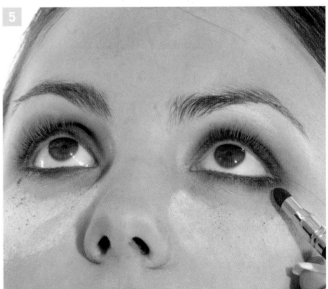

⑤ Apply the shadow on the lower lid close to the lashes and smudge with a blending brush or sponge into both inner and outer corners of the eye.

⑥ Apply a thick liquid line to the tops of the lids and extend the line to a feathered wisp at the outer corner of the eye. To really exaggerate the eyes apply either liquid or black pencil eyeliner to the inside corner of the eye and lower lids.

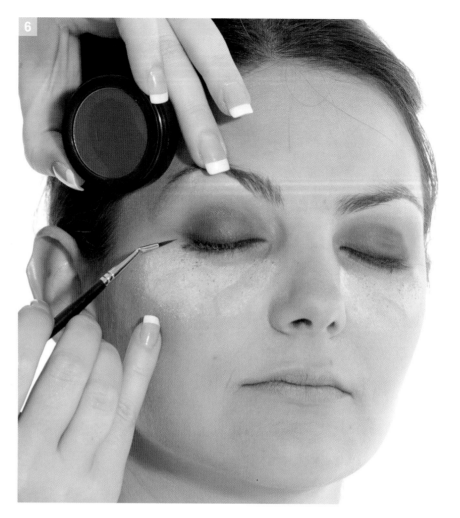

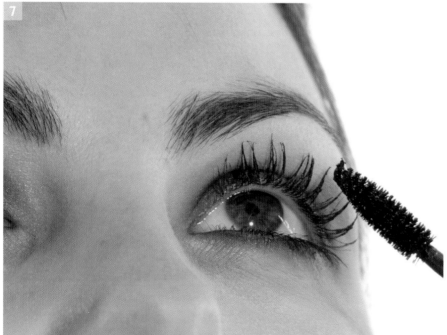

⑦ Apply lashings of mascara to the upper and lower lids, and for an even more spectacular result curl the lashes or add individual lash extensions to really perfect this look. For a hint of sparkle, coat the lashes with glitter mascara.

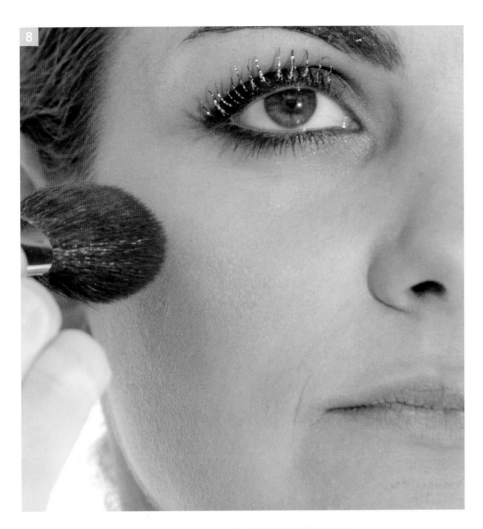

⑧ **A cream bronze or pink blush will complete the cheeks so blend into the apple of the cheeks and along the cheek bones.**

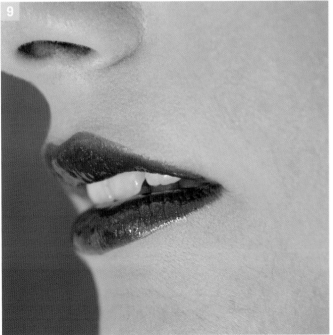

⑨ **To finish the look, choose a lipstick that complements the shadow colour you have chosen – deep colours look great with such heavy eyes. Use a pencil and matching lip product to enhance your natural features. In the 60s a very pale lip gloss was applied so for authenticity try this for an old twist! Gloss to finish will add shine and sexy sparkle to this look.**

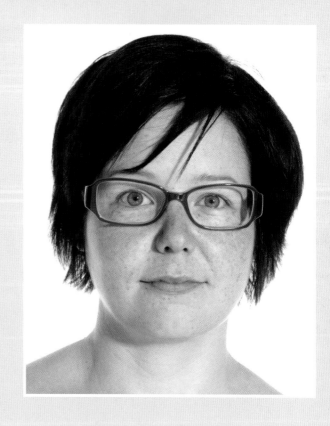

# dare to be bare

The 1980s were all about big hair, oversized shoulder pads and wild scary make-up! In the '90s we saw a range of diverse looks from vampy dark lips and eyes to sunblushed and natural, and whilst some of us would prefer to forget some of these elements of fashion we can appreciate their creative artistry. Some fantastic looks emerged from these years which have moulded present day looks.

See pages 146–147 for how to create this look

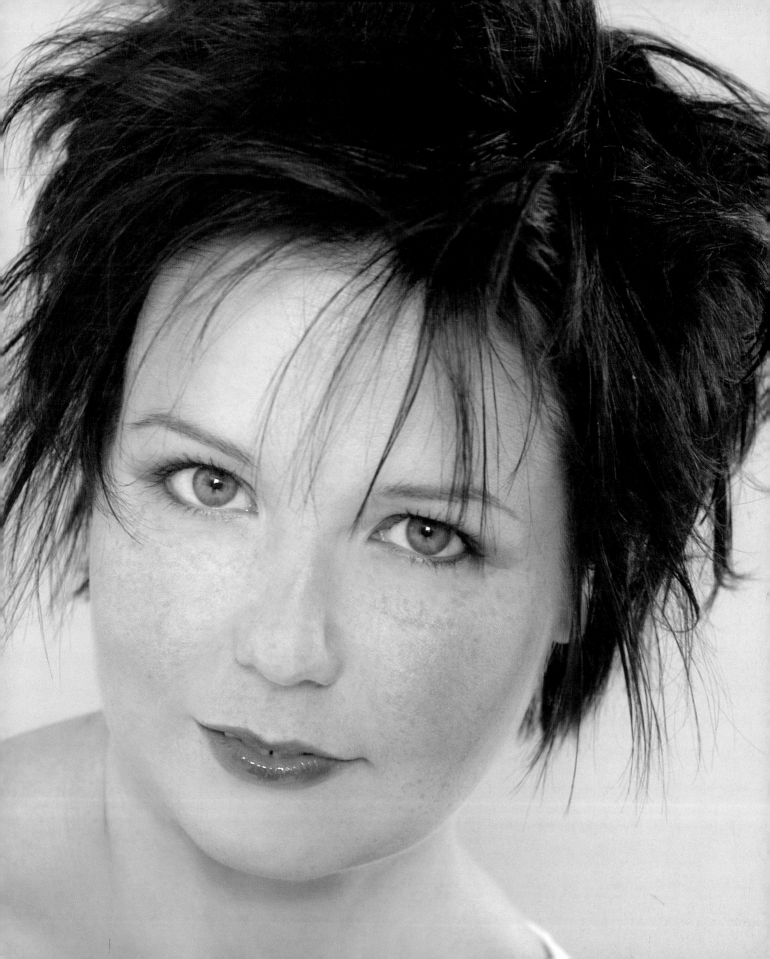

# how to...

## CREATE A DARE TO BE BARE LOOK

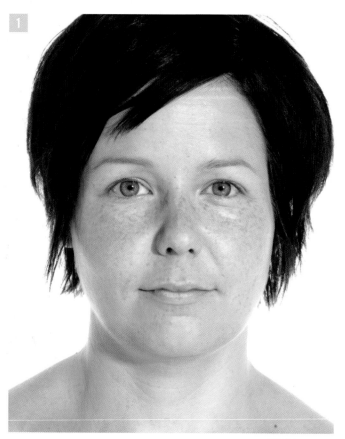

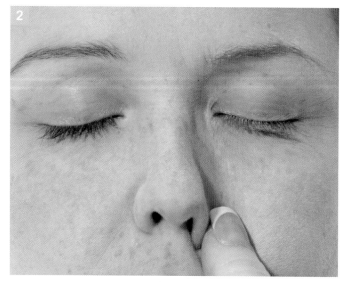

① The trick to a natural look is the foundation. Make this light and sheer to illuminate the skin and show your natural tones of flush.

③ Strip or individual lash extensions add glamour and a thin but lengthening coat of brown or black mascara will boost the depth of the eyes. For added depth pencil in brown or grey eyeliner to the outer corners of the top and bottom of the eyes and smudge with a liner sponge tool to give a smoky appearance.

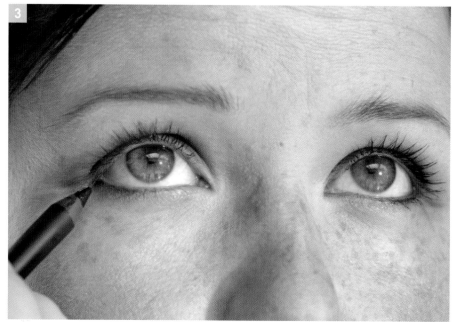

② Conceal under the eyes and around the nose using a wand concealer or chubby pencil to avoid the heaviness of a wax-based stick. Apply a champagne shadow with a shimmer to blend with the natural skin tones so that it covers the lids without being too noticeable. Use a white highlighter under the brows to accentuate and lift the eyes.

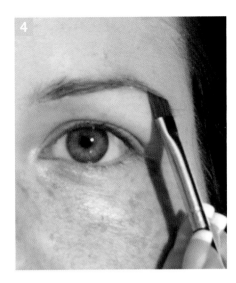

④ If the eyes are small, white eyeliner applied on the inside of the bottom lids will increase this natural look by widening the eyes. Very dark eyebrows can be bleached to lighten them to create a softer look or use a tawny coloured pencil or a brow brush and shadow to even out any gaps or unevenness of hair growth.

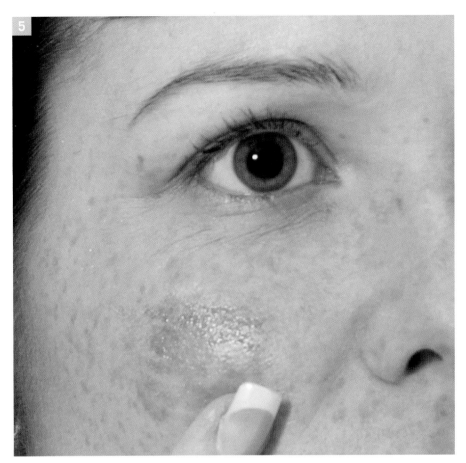

⑤ A cream blush or liquid will blend into the apple of the cheeks flawlessly and appear as a shimmer of peach or pink. Bronzers really only work on darker skins whereas pinks and peaches look fabulous on lighter complexions.

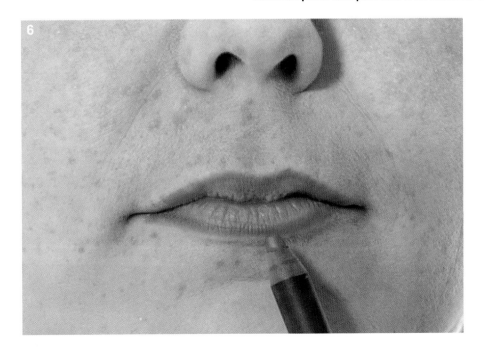

⑥ Line the lips with a neutral pink or very light brown then fill the lips with a sheer pink gloss to give a wet and very natural looking appearance.

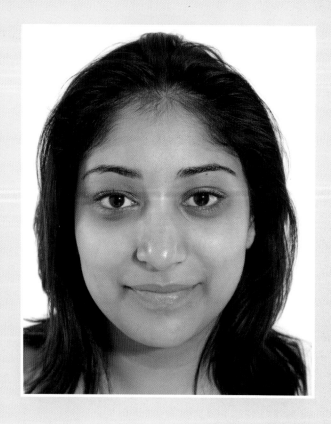

# metal mania

Glam rock and punk were seriously cool in the early 1980s
and metal looks with harsh lines and sparkles were very popular.
This look is always good for a party feel as well as if your really
want to show off your make-up talents!

See pages 150–151 for how to create this look

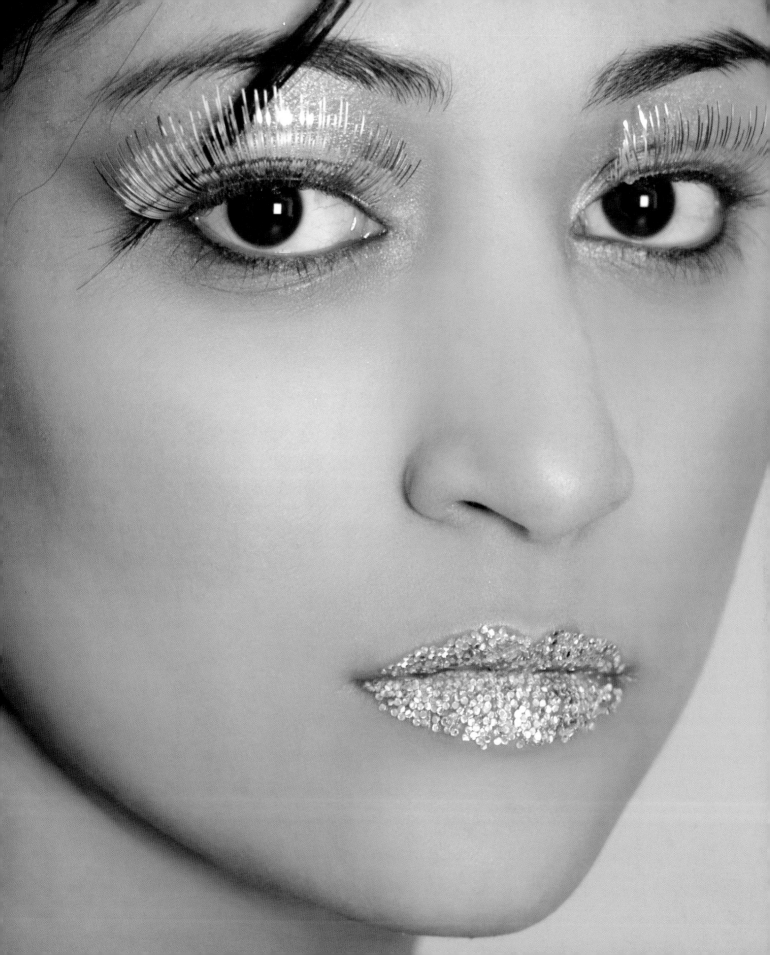

# how to...

## CREATE THE METAL MANIA LOOK

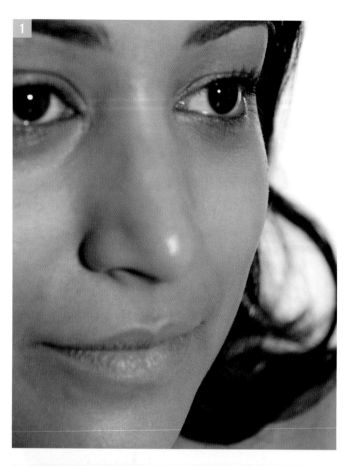

① Apply a foundation base to even out the skin tone and neutralise any irregular patches of colour. Conceal dark shadows and any tone differences with a liquid concealer.

② Blend a silver or gold base shadow on the lid up to the brows and apply a white highlighter under the brow to lift the eye colour and heighten the effect of this make-up. Using a shadow pencil or fine sponge, smooth a line of darker shadow or coloured shadow around the socket to add depth and breadth to the eyes.

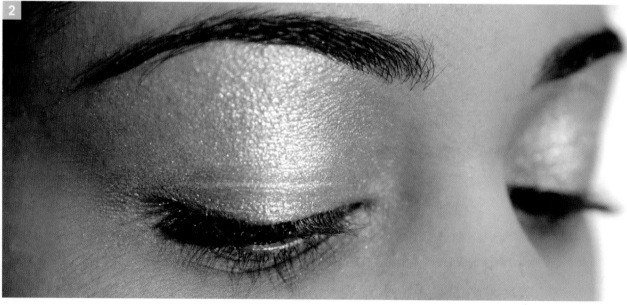

③ Glitz the brows with some glitter or simply a shimmer powder the same colour as the brow hairs. Add a touch of liquid shimmer to the top and bottom lids and false silver lashes to really vamp up this metallic look. You could simply use a coloured mascara instead for a more toned-down look.

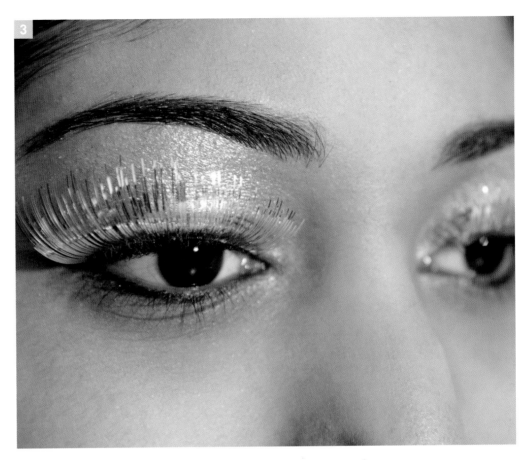

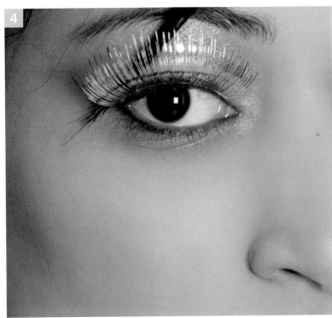

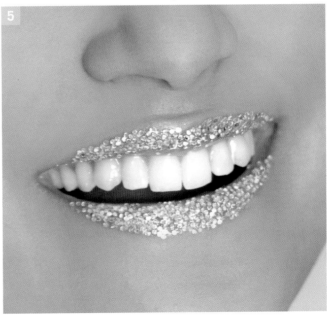

④ Blush the cheeks following the colour of your natural flush or if really daring try a silver shimmer! Add sparkle to the face by dusting over a shimmer powder.

⑤ Use a grey or copper lip liner to define the lips and then fill with a metallic lip shade or just pure glitter!

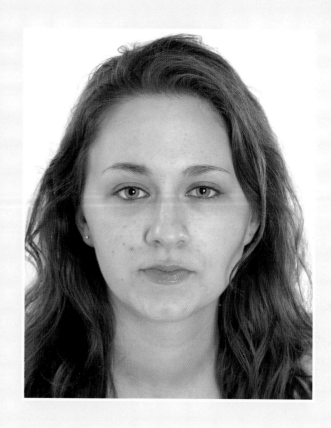

# nature's finest

In modern make-up there are no rules; you can experiment with colour, texture and style, and everything goes! Feel comfortable in what you wear and send onlookers a message that you are inventive, creative and wild at heart!

See pages 154–155 for how to create this look

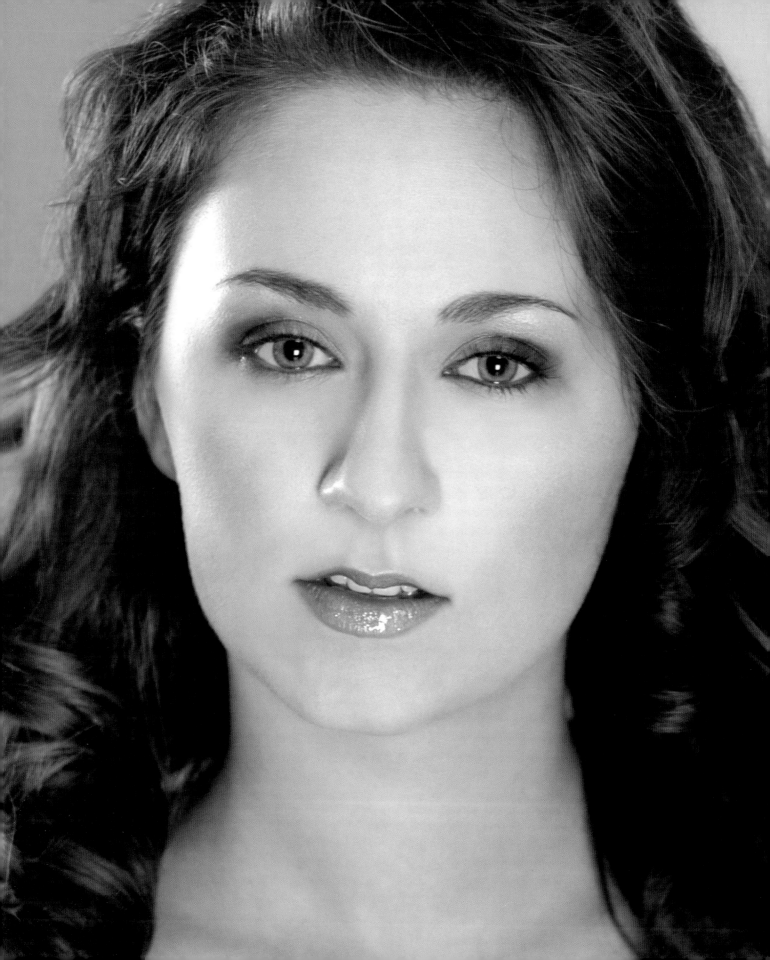

# how to...

## CREATE NATURE'S FINEST LOOK

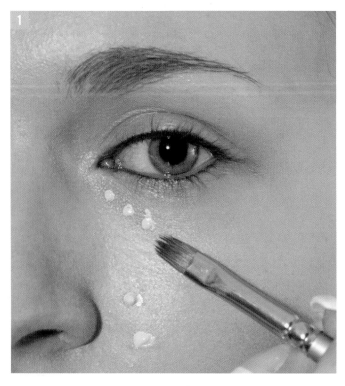

① Apply a sheer base of foundation with concealer to hide any blemishes, spots or dark patches of skin. Powder the base to secure it.

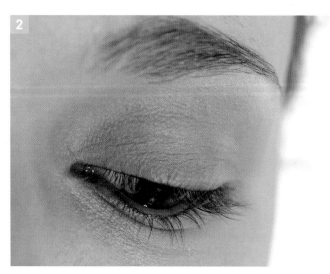

② Apply a light toned cream shadow on the socket up to the brows and blend thoroughly to ensure the whole eyelid is covered. This base canvas projects light onto the whole lid opening it up and making the eye appear larger.

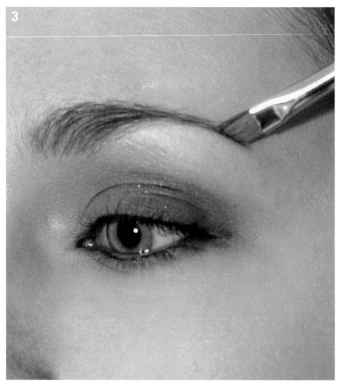

③ A white or paler shadow under the eyebrows to highlight the eyes will add depth. Block shadow the socket with a medium to dark shadow and blend to the edge of the socket only. Add a hint of earthy tone to the outer corner of the eye by using a green, deep copper, deep blue or grey. For extra enhancement carry on the colour to run under the lower lashes close to the root and smudge with the sponge or a cotton bud. Pencil the brows to define the colour and possibly give them a thicker more natural appearance. Brown or black mascara will lengthen and thicken the lashes whilst widening the eyes so add a double coat and comb through to remove any lumps.

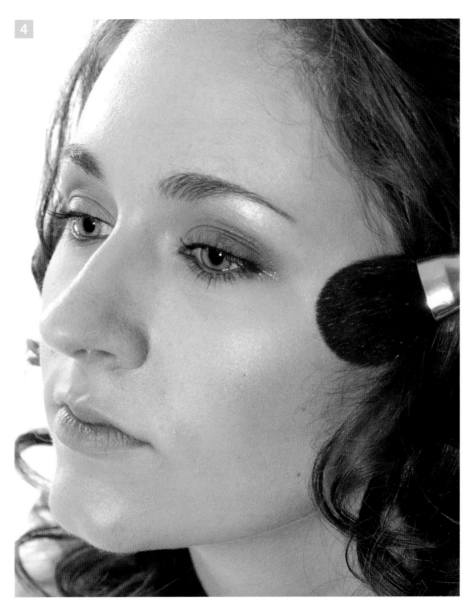

④ Shade the apple of the cheeks with a light pink shimmer and highlight the top of the apple with a shimmer powder or cream shimmer stick to give lustre and health to the cheeks.

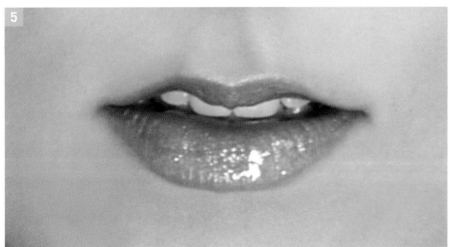

⑤ Line the lips with a medium brown liner and fill with either brown gloss or a natural shade matt lipstick. Add a touch of evening glitz by using shimmer, shine and glitter wherever possible!

# acknowledgements

I'd like to thank Steven Clennell and Anthony Braden Cosmetics for supplying such a wonderful array of inspiring make-up. Celine Bopp for her instinctive and wondrous make-up artistry for The Looks and the tireless models Charlotte and Charlotte, Rupi, Gray, Lorraine, Laura, Hanna, Taru, Lucy, Lisa, Alex and Colette for their patience and willingness to be adventurous! Thanks also to Paul West whose photography is truly an art in its own right. Also thanks to Corinne for editing out my bad jokes and to Rosemary for coming up with this wonderful idea in the first place.

Finally thanks to my family for their memories and ideas and to my long-suffering partner and best friend Elliot who will always be my true inspiration.

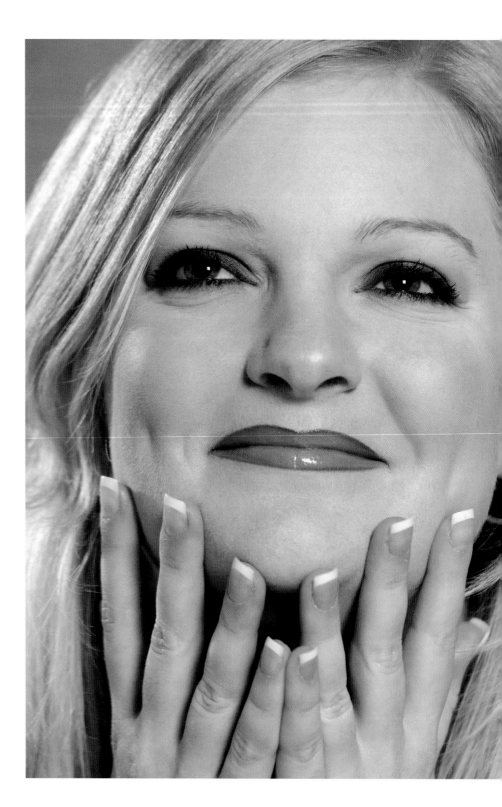

# index